Advances in Critical Care Testing

Springer

Berlin
Heidelberg
New York
Hong Kong
London
Milan
Paris
Tokyo

C. A. Burtis M. M. Müller (Eds.)

Advances in Critical Care Testing

The 2002 IFCC-Roche Diagnostics Award

Springer

Editors

Carl A. Burtis
Health Services Division
Oak Ridge National Laboratory
Oak Ridge TN 37831-6220
USA

Mathias M. Müller
Institute of Laboratory Diagnostics
Kaiser Franz Josef Hospital
Kundratstrasse 3
1100 Vienna, Austria

ISBN 3-540-40752-9 Springer-Verlag Berlin Heidelberg New York

Cataloging-in-Publication. Data applied for Bibliographic information published by Die Deutsche Bibliothek. Die Deutsche Bibliothek lists this publication in the Deutsche Nationalbibliografie; detailed bibliographic data ist available in the internet at http://dnb.ddb.de.
ISBN 3-540-40752-9

http://www.springer.de/medizin

Springer-Verlag Berlin Heidelberg 2004
Printed in Germany

Cover-Design: typographics GmbH, Darmstadt
Typesetting: typographics GmbH, Darmstadt

Printed on acid-free paper SPIN 10953747 18/5141 - 5 4 3 2 1 0 -

Table of Contents

List of Finalists XI

Preface XIII

Introduction XV

Heino von Prondzynski, Member of the Executive Committee of F. Hoffmann-La Roche AG and Head of the Diagnostics Division[1]

Winner of the 2002 IFCC-Roche Diagnostics Award

"Apoptosis In Sepsis And Multiple Organ Dysfunction Snydrome" 3
S. Zeerleder, B. Zwart, W. A. Wuillemin, L. A. Aarden, A. B. J. Groeneveld, C. Caliez, A. E. M. van Nieuwenhuijze; G. J. van Mierlo, A. J. M. Eerenberg, B. Lämmle, and C. E Hack

[1] These opening remarks were made on the occasion of the IFCC-Roche Diagnostics Award Presentation at the XVIII International Congress of Clinical Chemistry in Kyoto, Japan, October 22nd, 2002.

Inflammation – Infection – Sepsis

Finalists

"Plasma Procalcitonin And C-Reactive Protein In Acute Septic Shock: Clinical And Biological Correlates" ... 17
R. Claeys, S. Vinken, H. Spapen, K. ver Elst, L. Huyghens, F. K. Gorus

"Macrophage Migration Inhibitory Factor And Hypothalamo-Pituitary-Adrenal Function During Critical Illness" ... 32
A. Beishuizen, L. J. Thijs, C. Haanen, I. N. Vermes

"Early Identification Of High Risk Critically Ill Patients And Comparison With Acute Physiology Scores For Predicting Outcome" ... 47
M. Manji, P. Gosling, and S. Brudney

National Winners

"4G/5G Promoter Polymorphism In The Plasminogen Activator Inhibitor-1 Gene In Children With Systemic Meningococcaemia" ... 65
G. Geishofer, W. Zenz, B. Resch, S. Panzer, G. Endler, D. Häring, C. Mannhalter

"Quantification Of Viral Genomes In Immunocompromised Patients" ... 69
B. M. Halima, Z. Arrouji, H. Dhaouadi, A. Slim, E. Ben Hassen, T. Ben Chaabane, S. Ben Redjeb

"Haptoglobin Polymorphism And Mortality In Patients With Tuberculosis" ... 72
I. Kasvosve, Z. A. R. Gomo, E. Mvundura, V. M. Moyo, T. Saungweme, H. Khumalo, V. R. Gordeuk, J. R. Boelaert, J. R. Delanghe, D. De Bacquer, I. T. Gangaidzo

Hypoxia – Ischaemia

Finalist

"Phospholipases A_2 Levels And Distribution In Bronchoalveolar Lavage Fluid Of Patients With Acute Respiratory Distress Syndrome (ARDS): Application Of A Fluorimetric Method" ... 77
E. I. Kitsiouli, G. Nakos, M. E. Lekka

Blood Gases – Electrolytes – Trace Elements

National Winner

"Magnesium In The ICU" 93
A. Abraham, A. Bachwani

Cardiology – Haemodynamics – Stroke

Finalist

"Single-Point Troponin T Measurement On The Day Of Coronary Care Unit Discharge After Myocardial Infarction Strongly Correlates With Ejection Fraction And Infarct Size By Nuclear Imaging And With CK-MB Release" 97
G. Bonetti, F. Pagani, R. Giubbini, C. Cuccia, M. Panteghini

National Winner

"Soluble Adhesion Molecules In Acute Stroke" 111
A. M. Simundic, V. Basic, E. Topic, V. Demarin, N. Vrkic, B. Kunovic, M. Stefanovic, A. Begonja

Nephrology

National Winner

"Monitoring Of The Renal Functions During Continuous Renal Replacement Therapy – The Application Of The Analysis Of Cystatin C And Natriuretic Peptides" 115
M. Balik, A. Jabor, A. Hendl, M. Koláø, M. Pavlisová, D. Brestan

Haematology – Haemostatis

National Winners

"Serum Levels Of Soluble Transferrin Receptors (sTfR) Correlate Better With Severity Of Disease Than With Iron Stores In Patients With Malignant Lymphomas" 119
J. Bjerner, L. M. Amlie, L. S. Rusten, E. Jakobsen

"The Functional Activity Of Platelets In Surgery Patients With Artificial Cardiac Valve" ... 120
T. Lobachevskaya, T. Vavilova, M. Kadinskaya, D. Polezhaev

"Serum Oxidative State Followng Thrombolysis Combined With ABCIXIMAB In Comparison To r-PA Or Streptokinase Alone" ... 122
I. Maor, G. Slobodin, E. Goldhammer, S. Shnizer, T. Kagan, E. G. Abinader, A. Lanir

New Technology – Methods

Finalists

"A Rapid And Sensitive Immunoassay For Determination Of S-100 Protein In A Point-Of-Care Setting" ... 127
S. Eriksson, L. Dean, K. Pettersson

"Plasma DNA As A Noninvasive Monitoring Tool For Trauma Patients" ... 142
Y. M. D. Lo, T. H. Rainer

"Clinical Application Of A Highly Sensitive Immuno-Polymerase Chain Reaction For Serum Tumor Necrosis Factor α" ... 154
D. Kobayashi, K. Saito, M. Komatsu, N. Watanabe

"Rapid And Reliable Detection Of Fungemia By Polymerase Chain Reaction" ... 163
U. H. Tirodker, J. P. Nataro, K. D. Fairchild

National Winner

"A New Approach Of Endotoxin Testing By Using A Monoclonal Antibody Against Endotoxin (WN1-222/5) And Flow Cytometry" ... 177
J. Nolde, F. E. Di Padova, H. Brade H., K. H. Staubach

Organizational Aspects

National Winner

"Improvement Of Critical Care Management In A Healthcare Area By Implementing Point-Of-Care Testing In Primary Care. A Preliminary Approach" 183
M. L. Hortas, I. Pérez-Montaut, M. Redondo, N. Montiel, R. Molina, C. González

Miscellaneous

National Winners

"Studies On The Potential Effect Of Nitrite" 187
Y. Tian, C. Wang, S. Song

"Evaluation Of Some Laboratory Abnormalities In Acute Opiate Intoxication" 189
H. T. Hung

"Adhesion Molecules In An In Vitro Model Of Graft Rejection" 192
S. Markovič, H. Daxecker, Ì. Raab, A. Griesmacher, M. M. Müller

Index 195

About Roche and the Roche Diagnostics Division 199

List of Finalists

Dr. Graziella Bonetti
Spedali Civili – Brescia
U.O. Laboratorio Analisi Chimico Cliniche 1
Piazzale Spedali Civili, 1
25125 Brescia
Italy

Bert Beishuizen MD PhD
Internist-intensivist
Department of Intensive Care 7D118
VU University Medical Center
PO Box 7057
1007 MB Amsterdam
Netherlands

Prof. Dr. YM Dennis Lo
Department of Chemical Pathology
Room 38023
1/F Clinical Sciences Building
Prince of Wales Hospital
30–32 Ngan Shing Street
Shatin, New Territories
Hong Kong

Dr. Daisuke Kobayashi
VA Medical Center
Bldg 3, Rm. 2B102
1400 VFW Parkway
West Roxbury, MA 02132
USA

Dr. med. S. Zeerleder
Spitalzentrum Biel
Innere Medizin
Im Vogelsang 84
2502 Biel
Switzerland

Dr. Roxane Claeys
Regionaal Ziekenhuis H. Hart
Clinical Laboratory
Naamsestraat 105
3000 Leuven
Belgium

Dr. Urmila Tirodker
Childrens Hospital Medical Center of Akron
Division of Critical Care
One Perkins Square
Akron, Ohio 44308-1062
USA

Dr. Susann Eriksson
Department of Biotechnology
University of Turku
Tykistökatu 6 A, 6th floor
20520 Turku
Finland

Dr. Eirini Kitsiouli
Lab. Biochemistry
Chemistry Dept.
University of Ioannina
T.K. 45100
Ioannina
Greece

Dr. Mav Manji
University Hospital Birmingham NHS Trust
Selly Oak Critical Care (SOCC)
Raddlebarn Road
Selly Oak
Birmingham B29 6JD
United Kingdom

Preface

The IFCC-Roche Diagnostics Award for Advances in Critical Care Testing was established in 1996 to encourage and recognize young scientists who are carrying out research and development in the area of critical care testing.

The organization of the award is based on a three-year cycle which initially involves competition at a national level followed by an international final. The applicants for the 2002 IFCC-Roche Diagnostics Award came from 34 member countries of the IFCC. The papers and abstracts covered a wide range of topics relating to the development, application and interpretation of new or existing tests for diagnosis, monitoring and treatment of critically ill patients. The National Societies of the IFCC were responsible for the selection of the National Winner in each country and the IFCC-Roche Diagnostics Award Committee then selected 10 finalists from the national winners to present their work in a special Symposium convened at the Kyoto International Congress of Clinical Chemistry and Laboratory Medicine in October of 2002. From these 10 finalists, **Dr. Sacha Zeerleder** from the Central Hematology Laboratory, University Hospital, Bern Switzerland and the Central Laboratory of the Netherlands Red Cross Blood Transfusion Service, Amsterdam, the Netherlands was selected as the winner of the competition for his paper entitled "Apoptosis In Sepsis And Multiple Organ Dysfunction Syndrome". At the Awards Ceremony he was presented with a certificate and a cheque for US$ 30 000.

This book is the third volume of Advances in Critical Care Testing and it contains the ten papers from the final ten contestants with abstracts from some of the other participants in the competition. In addition, we have included an address made by Heino von Prondzynski, Member of the Executive Committee of F. Hoffmann-La Roche AG and Head of the Diagnostics Division on the occasion of the Awards Ceremony of the Kyoto Congress.

As the title of this volume indicates, all the major fields of intensive care and emergency medicine are represented. This includes stress, inflammation, infection, hypoxia, ischaemia, cardiology, haemodynamics, nephrology, haematology, blood gases, electrolytes and trace elements as well as new developments in laboratory practice such as the application of molecular biology.

The editors would like to express their appreciation to all the National Societies of IFCC who promoted this Award amongst their members and selected their National Winners. In addition we must thank our fellow members of the IFCC-Roche Diagnostics Awards Committee who selected the ten finalists and then had the very difficult task of selecting the winner of the 2002 Award.

This award was initially known as the IFCC-AVL Awards as it was created by the IFCC and AVL with AVL sponsoring the 1996 and 1999 competitions. With its acquisition of AVL, Roche Diagnostics assumed sponsorship of the 2002 award as an indication of their commitment to fostering interdisciplinary research and development in the area of critical care testing. On behalf of the IFCC we would like to express our sincere thanks to AVL for their initial support and involvement and to Roche Diagnostics for their continuing and generous support. Apart from the prize money and travel support, Roche Diagnostics has provided considerable time in organising the Award and to publishing this book. We would especially like to acknowledge the invaluable and reliable assistance of Ildikó Amann-Zalán from Roche Diagnostics for her dedication and perseverance in keeping the award on schedule.

We are confident that you will find the research contained within the following pages both interesting and stimulating. We look forward to receiving applications for the next IFCC-Roche Diagnostics Award, the final of which, will take place in 2005 at the ICCC in Orlando, Florida.

Carl A. Burtis, Oak Ridge Tennessee, USA and
Mathias M. Müller, Vienna, Austria

Introduction

Heino von Prondzynski, Member of the Executive Committee of F. Hoffmann-La Roche AG and Head of the Diagnostics Division[2]

"Ladies and Gentlemen,

I would like to welcome you to the ceremony of the 3rd IFCC-Roche Diagnostics Award during the International Congress of Clinical Chemistry and Laboratory Medicine here in Kyoto. A special compliment goes to the members of the jury, Professor Carl Burtis, Professor Ann Gronowski, Professor Adolf Grünert, Professor Werner List, Professor James Nichols and Professor John Whitfield, the finalists, all IFCC members, represented by its President Professor Mathias Müller and to my colleagues from Roche Diagnostics. Without the outstanding dedication from all of you this Award could not have been made such a success. I would also like to thank our Japanese hosts who have organized this international congress in the beautiful environment of Kyoto.

It is an honor and a great pleasure for me today to award together with our partner, the IFCC, the scientist or clinician who has developed the most significant advances in the area of critical care testing. The intention of the IFCC-Roche Diagnostics Award is to encourage and recognize young scientists who are carrying out research and development for a clinical or laboratory improvement related to critically ill patients. The results of this award will help to further improve the treatment of those patients and save lives.

Why are awards like this important? Diagnostics and medicine will be undergoing a revolutionary change during the years to come. Medicine will focus much more on treating causes and not simply symptoms. The importance of diagnostics will increase substantially from diagnosis and treatment monitoring to preposition screening, targeted monitoring and prevention of diseases.

Genomics and proteomics will allow us completely new insights into the human body. The map of the human genome, which has been done only to some extend yet, will open us a huge potential of further health information and how to prevent and manage diseases and live healthier. Based on this broad knowledge it will be the future challenge to all of us to create true innovation out of this. We will not have a lack of information, in contrast it will be much more than a single person

[2] These opening remarks were made on the occasion of the IFCC-Roche Diagnostics Award Presentation at the XVIII International Congress of Clinical Chemistry in Kyoto, Japan, October 22nd, 2002

can oversee, but we will have a huge need to use this information in the most effective way. We want to pioineer integrated and individualized solutions so that the next generation will know some of today's diseases only from hearsay.

As the world's No. 1 in-vitro Diagnostic Company, we recognize our unique responsibility to the health care community and all people who want to live a healthier life. Research & Development have always been and will be a fundamental pillar of our industry. We at Roche Diagnostics want new ideas to flourish within our labs and research teams. Therefore we are not only spending about 10 per cent of the total sales for R&D every year, but also initiated an internal venture process two years ago. Our goal is to exploit new areas and learn in fields others haven't done or even might have thought of. Having the opportunity to act as an entrepreneur and work with transnational teams, without baring the financial risk of a start-up, makes this so interesting for our employees.

But to meet the challenges of the future we additionally need to share ideas and know-how within the industry, where we set up alliances, and with the scientific community. We want to support young scientist and researchers and help them to make their solutions better known and to be implemented. This award can be seen as a sign for a cooperation between industry and science. If we are able to maintain a steady transfer of know-how between us we will all profit.

It is the third time this award has been posted and we are proud that it has achieved growing interest amongst the target groups. Since the acquisition of AVL Medical Instruments, Roche Diagnostics plays a much more active role in the field of critical care testing. We are a leading supplier in the fields of coagulation monitoring as well as blood gas and electrolyte analyzers at the most critical points. And we want to strengthen our expertise further. An example, which came out of the before mentioned venture process, was the so-called "PCR meets ICU" venture. The solution found by our employees replaces serological applications with PCR technology for rapid sepsis testing. This cuts testing time from days to hours, which is a life saving factor in case a sepsis occurs.

We are looking forward to further develop this area together with the applicants of the award. This time, 71 scientists and clinicians from 34 countries all over the world have sent in their applications showing a high standard. The ten best papers have been selected from the group of the national winners and finally, out of these ten one had to be chosen. I think the jury will completely agree with me – it was no easy choice.

We have received very interesting and promising abstracts with a high standard and it has been difficult to choose one as "the best one" – because all of them are great in their dedication and their commitment to improve diagnostic tools in critical care units. Awarding one winner does not mean that the other improvements are less important for patients. I would like to thank all of you very much for your innovative spirit and your enthusiasm – people like you are the fundamental basis on which our health care systems can improve day by day. Congratulations to all of you."

WINNER of the 2002 IFCC-ROCHE DIAGNOSTICS AWARD

Apoptosis In Sepsis And Multiple Organ Dysfunction Syndrome

S. Zeerleder, B. Zwart, W. A. Wuillemin, L. A. Aarden, A. B. J. Groeneveld, C. Caliez, A. E. M. van Nieuwenhuijze; G. J. van Mierlo, A. J. M. Eerenberg, B. Lämmle, and C. E. Hack

Central Hematology Laboratory, University Hospital, Bern, SWITZERLAND
Central Laboratory of the Netherlands Red Cross Blood Transfusion Service, Amsterdam, the NETHERLANDS

Key words:
Sepsis, MODS, apoptosis, nucleosome

Abstract

Introduction

Multiple organ dysfunction syndrome (MODS) is a frequent complication of severe sepsis and septic shock. Although massive inflammatory reaction is considered to be one of the main triggers for the development of MODS, outcome is not necessarily improved by blocking the action of these mediators. Therefore, the downstream effects of these inflammatory mediators, such as the induction of apoptosis, might be pivotal in the pathogenesis of MODS. However, only indirect markers for apoptosis, such as soluble FAS, can be measured in plasma. During the later stages of apoptosis, nucleosomes are released from cell's chromatin by internucleosomal cleavage by endonucleases. We investigated whether circulating nucleosomes constitute a marker for apoptosis in sepsis.

Methods

We assessed circulating levels of nucleosomes, specific markers released by cells during the later stages of apoptosis, with a previously described ELISA in plasma of 69 patients suffering from fever (n=14), systemic inflammatory response syndrome (SIRS; n=15), severe sepsis (n=32) or septic shock (n=8). Severity of MODS was assessed with sepsis scores, clinical and laboratory parameters.

Results

Elevated nucleosome levels were found in 64%, 60%, 94% and 100% of patients suffering from fever, SIRS, severe sepsis or septic shock, respectively. In patients with advanced MODS, nucleosome levels correlated well with cytokine plasma levels (Interleukin-6 and -8) as well as with parameters predictive for outcome (Plasminogen activator type-1, C3a).

Significantly higher nucleosome levels in patients with septic shock than in patients with severe sepsis ($p=0.038$), SIRS ($p=0.0033$) and fever ($p<0.0001$), respectively. Significantly higher nucleosome levels in patients with severe sepsis than in patients with SIRS ($p=0.002$) and with fever ($p<0.0001$), respectively. Comparison between groups was performed by using Mann-Whitney Rank Sum Test. SIRS: Systemic inflammatory response syndrome.

Conclusion

Patients with severe sepsis and septic shock have elevated plasma levels of nucleosomes. We suggest that apoptosis, probably resulting from exposure of cells to excessive amounts of inflammatory mediators, is crucial in the pathogenesis of MODS.

Introduction

Despite advances in supportive therapy and the use of potent antibiotics, mortality rates of patients suffering from severe sepsis have not impressively improved over the past 20 years. At present, sepsis is a major cause of death with a mortality up to 50% in intensive care units (ICU) (1). Multiple organ dysfunction syndrome (MODS) is a frequent complication of severe sepsis and septic shock contributing to the high mortality. Although massive inflammatory responses likely are main triggers of MODS, outcome is not necessarily improved by blocking the action of these inflammatory mediators (2,3). Therefore, the downstream effects of inflammatory mediators might be pivotal in the pathogenesis of MODS. A potential downstream effect is widespread cellular apoptosis in various organs, which may lead to organ dysfunction. Apoptosis or programmed cell death is, in contrast to necrosis, an active suicidal cellular response involved in the homeostasis of cell removal under physiological and pathological conditions (3). Indeed, various observations support a role for increased apoptosis in the development of MODS. In a sepsis model in mice, apoptosis of lymphocytes and parenchymal cells in various organs was found (4). Increased liver cell apoptosis in mice was reduced by administration of anti-TNF-á antibodies (5). Also, in clinical sepsis there is indirect evidence for an increased rate of cellular apoptosis. Patients with sepsis and MODS have elevated levels of soluble Fas (sFas), which decrease when MODS improves (6). Nuclear matrix protein (NMP), a general marker for cell death not specifically indicating apoptosis was shown to correlate with MODS-scores and disease severity (7). In patients suffering from abdominal sepsis, increased plasma cell apoptosis was detected in the mucosa of the small intestine (8). Thus, apoptosis is likely involved in the pathogenesis of sepsis. However, in humans only indirect markers for apoptosis (e.g. sFas) were assessed until now.

Cytoplasmic and chromatin condensation, and nuclear fragmentation are the morphologic features of apoptosis. Nuclear fragmentation results in a characteristic pattern of a DNA-ladder of 180 basepairs (bp) in agarose gel electrophoresis, and results from chromatin degradation by endonucleases (9). These enzymes cleave DNA between so-called nucleosomes, which are core particles composed of an octamer of 2 copies each of histones H2A, H2B, H3 and H4, around which a stretch of helical DNA of 146 bp length is wrapped (10). Cells release nucleosomes during the later stages of apoptosis. These nucleosomes can be measured in plasma and therefore constitute a soluble parameter for apoptosis (van Nieuwenhuijze et al., manuscript submitted).

To investigate the role of apoptosis in the pathogenesis of sepsis and MODS, we measured plasma levels of nucleosomes in patients suffering from fever, systemic inflammatory response syndrome (SIRS), severe sepsis or septic-shock.

Material and Methods

Patients

Patients of the medical and surgical wards or Intensive Care Units (ICU) were eligible if they had fever, or met the inclusion criteria for SIRS, severe sepsis or septic shock. Fever was defined as axillar or rectal temperature of ≥ 38°C and ≥ 38.3°C, respectively (11). The diagnosis of SIRS, severe sepsis and septic shock was established according to the definitions of the ACCP consensus conference (12). In addition, the following definitions were used: hypotension: systolic blood pressure < 90mmHg or a drop in systolic blood pressure of ≥ 40 mmHg for more than 1 hour in the presence of adequate fluid substitution and the absence of antihypertensive agents. Renal insufficiency: either urinary output < 0.5 ml/kg body weight per hour, or < 30 ml per 2 hours, or serum creatinine > 180 µmol/L (2 mg/dl), or an elevation to more than two times the baseline serum creatinine level despite adequate fluid replacement therapy, or new need for dialysis. Lactic acidosis: level of serum lactate > 2.2 mmol/L together with a pH of < 7.3 or a base excess value of < –10 mmol/L. Central nervous system impairment: Glasgow Coma Scale (GCS) of < 11 points or a drop of > 2 points compared to the baseline value. Liver insufficiency: the presence of at least two of the following criteria: total bilirubin level > 43 µmol/l; aspartate aminotransferase or alanine aminotransferase levels more than two times the normal value; activated partial thromboplastin time > 1.5 times the normal value (13).

The clinical evaluation of patients with fever and SIRS included in this study was described in detail elsewhere (11). Patients suffering from severe sepsis or septic shock were followed for 90 days or until death. In these latter patients, the logistic organ dysfunction (LOD) score (14) and sepsis-related organ failure assessment

(SOFA) score (15) were calculated at entry. The principle of both score systems is to characterize the degree of dysfunction of 6 organ systems by a point system including the cardiovascular, pulmonary, neurologic, renal, hematologic and hepatic system. The range of point scores varies from 0 to 22 in the LOD score and from 0 to 24 points in the SOFA score. Diagnostic investigations of suspected foci of infection (e.g. cultures of blood and tissue) were done according to the decisions of the attending physician. The 32 patients suffering from severe sepsis and 8 suffering from septic shock participated in a randomized, double blind, placebo-controlled pilot trial to study the efficacy and safety of C1-inhibitor (C1-Inh) substitution in severe sepsis and septic shock. Twenty patients received C1-Inh, 20 recieved placebo. The 28-day and 90-day mortality was 25% and 32%, respectively, with no difference between C1-Inh and placebo group. The 28-day mortality in 8 patients suffering from septic shock was 50%. Except for one patient in the treatment group, who died from an intra-operative aortic rupture, all patients demised due to the septic process.

Blood collection

Arterial blood was collected on admission for cytokine and complement analysis in vials containing EDTA (4 mM K_2EDTA [final concentration], Sarstedt Monovette®, Nürnbrecht, Germany). For the determination of the clotting factors, citrate-containing vials (1 part of 0.106 M Na_3citrate; Sarstedt Monovette®; 9 parts of blood) were used.

Plasma was prepared by centrifuging blood vials twice at room temperature for 10 min each at 1500xg, and stored in small aliquots in polypropylene tubes at –70°C until analysis

Laboratory analyses

Routine parameters: Routine hematologic, chemistry and coagulation parameters were obtained at study entry.

Nucleosome ELISA: Nucleosome levels were assessed with a recently developed ELISA (Nieuwenhuijze et al., manuscript submitted). In this ELISA, monoclonal antibody CLB-ANA/58 (CLB, Amsterdam, the Netherlands), which recognizes an epitope exposed on complexes of histone 2A, histone 2B and dsDNA, present only on nucleosomes, was used as a detecting antibody. Monoclonal antibody CLB-ANA/60 which reacts with histone 3, was used as the catching antibody. Briefly, microtitre plates were coated at 4°C overnight with 2 μg/ml mAb CLB-ANA/60 in 0.05 M carbonate buffer (pH 9.6). After 5 washes with phosphate buffered saline (PBS)-0.02% (w/v) Tween 20 (PT), samples were diluted in High Performance ELISA-buffer (HPE-buffer, CLB) containing 0.1 M sodium EDTA (pH 8.4) and 5% (v/v) DNAse-I-treated normal mouse serum and incubated for 60 minutes at room temperature. After 5 washes with PT, wells were incubated with 0.5 µg/ml biotinylated mAb CLB-ANA/58 (CLB) in PBS followed for 60 minutes at room temperature. Plates were washed 5 times with PT, and streptavidin-polymerized horse radish peroxidase (poly-HRP; CLB) diluted 10.000 times in HPE-buffer was added for 20 minutes. After washing 5 times with PT, plates were developed by adding 100 mg/ml 3,3',5,5'-Tetramethylbenzidin (TMB, Merck, Darmstadt, Germany) and 0.003% (v/v) hydrogen-peroxide in 0.11 M sodium acetate buffer (pH 5.5) for 5 min, and the reaction stopped by adding 2 M H_2SO_4. Absorbance was measured at 450 nm. As a standard, supernatant of apoptotic Jurkat cells was used. This supernatant was prepared by incubating Jurkat cells with 200 µM etoposide for one week to induce apoptosis. The supernatant was collected and stored in aliquots of approximately 1 ml at −70°C. Plasma levels were expressed as U/ml. One unit was arbitrarily set at the amount of nucleosomes released by 100 Jurkat cells. Levels of nucleosomes in healthy persons are undetectable, i.e. < 35 U/ml.

Cytokines: Plasma concentrations of TNF-α, IL-6, IL-8, and IL-10 were measured with ELISA's previously described (16,17). Values were given in pg/ml.

Statistical analysis

Results are expressed as median with range. Statistical analysis was performed using a commercial statistical package (SigmaStatÓ, Jandel, San Rafael, CA). The Mann-Whitney Rank Sum Test was used to assess differences between groups at a given time. Correlations between parameters were assessed by using Spearman's Rank Correlation. Statistical significance was considered as $p < 0.05$.

Results

Patients

Sixty-nine patients were enrolled in the study: 14 with fever, 15 with SIRS, 32 suffering from severe sepsis and 8 from septic shock. Eight of the patients in both the fever as well as the SIRS group were females. The median age in these groups were 60 [range: 27–92] and 65 [38–77] years, respectively. Among the 32 patients with severe sepsis, 7 were females (median age: 69 years [range 50–74]) and 25 males (64 years [28–74]). All 8 patients enrolled with septic shock were males (52 years [29–74]). Laboratory baseline parameters in patients suffering from severe sepsis and septic shock are given in table 1.

Table 1. Laboratory baseline characteristics in patients with severe sepsis and septic shock

	Severe sepsis (n=32)		Septic shock (n=8)	
	median	range	median	range
Hb (g/l)	94.5*	76.0–129.0	118.0*	88.0–145.0
Lc (x10⁹/l)	11.6	2.4–24.0	9.7	1.5–24.6
Tc (x10⁹/l)	179.0*	38.0–484.0	56.5*	7.0–334.0
Creat (µmol/L)	115.0	67.0–717.0	287.0	81.0–444.0
ASAT (U/l)	37.0	6.0–1865.0	63.5	26.0–3340.0
ALAT (U/l)	23.0	5.0–438.0	37.5	7.0–1380.0
CRP (mg/l)	211.5	4.0–444.0	158.5	41.0–396.0
LOD score	4.5	1.0–10.0	5.0	2.0–14.0
SOFA score	8.0	5.0–14.0	12.0	4.0–18.0

Abbreviations: Hb: hemoglobin, Lc: leukocytes, Tc: thrombocytes, Creat: creatinine, ASAT: aspartate aminotransferase, ALAT: alanine aminotransferase, CRP: C-reactive protein, LOD score: logistic organ dysfunction score, SOFA score: sepsis-related organ failure assessment score. * indicates statistically significant difference ($p<0.05$) between the 2 groups.

Nucleosome plasma levels

Elevated nucleosome levels were found in 56 (81%) of the 69 patients studied. The proportion of patients with elevated levels of nucleosomes increased with increasing severity of the inflammatory condition: 64% and 60% of the patients with fever or SIRS, respectively, 94% of those with severe sepsis, and 100% of the septic shock patients (figure 1). Comparison of absolute levels revealed higher values in the patients with more severe disease. The septic shock patients had significantly higher nucleosome levels (median [range]: 814 U/ml [52–1979]) than those with severe sepsis (269 U/ml [<35–1947]), SIRS (53 U/ml [<35–793]) or fever (38 U/ml [<35–285]), respectively, ($p<0.05$). Similarly, nucleosome levels in patients with severe sepsis were significantly higher than those in patients with SIRS or fever, and they tended to be higher in the patients with SIRS as compared to those with fever alone.

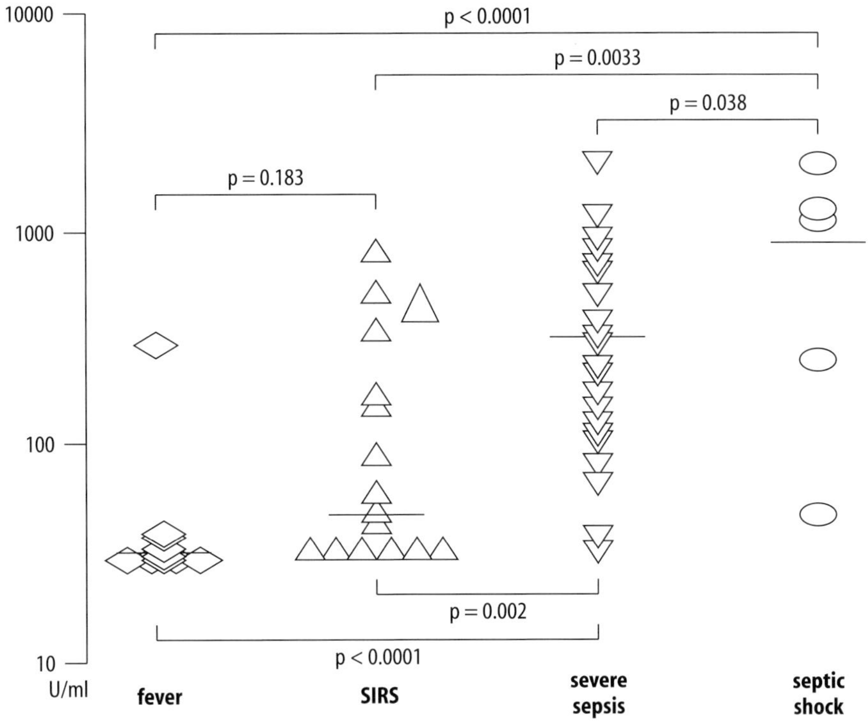

Legend: patients with fever (n=14) ◇; with SIRS (n=15) △, with severe sepsis (n=32) ▽, or with septic shock (n=8) ○. indicates median values for each group. —

Figure 1. Nucleosome levels in patients with fever, SIRS, severe sepsis and septic shock. Nucleosome levels between patients with severe sepsis and fever or SIRS are significant (p<0.0001 and p=0.002, respectively). Differences in nucleosome levels between the group with septic shock and fever or SIRS are significant (p<0.0001 and p=0.0033, respectively). Nucleosome levels between patients with severe sepsis and septic shock are significantly different (p=0.038). Normal persons have undetectable levels(<35U/ml).

In 72.5 % of the 40 patients suffering from severe sepsis or septic shock, the infecting microorganism was identified. Infections with gram-negative or gram-positive organisms, or double infections occurred in 22.5% (n=9), 27.5% (n=11), and 12.5% (n=5), respectively. Nucleosome levels did not differ between these groups. Four patients had a infections with Parainfluenza-virus (type-1), Mycoplasma pneumoniae, bacillus Calmette-Guérin (BCG) or Candida albicans, respectively. These patients were not considered separately. Eleven patients had no detectable infecting microorganism. Nucleosome levels in these patients were comparable to those in patients with identified infection.

Relation of nucleosome levels to mortality and other parameters

Nucleosome levels in non-surviving patients (with severe sepsis or septic shock (n=13) tended to be higher (628 U/ml [<35–1979]) than those in survivors (n=27; 276 U/ml [<35–1947]), although this level did not reach statistical significance (p=0.333). With increasing severity of organ dysfunction, nucleosome levels correlated better with cytokines, complement, coagulation and fibrinolytic parameters as well as with activation markers for neutrophils. Correlations in patients with a LOD- and SOFA-score of ≥ 6 and ≥ 12, respectively, are given in table 2. At a LOD-score ≥ 6 (n=11), IL-6, IL-8 and IL-10 correlated positively (r > 0.5) with nucleosome levels. At a SOFA score ≥ 9 (n=16), IL-6 levels correlated significantly with nucleosome levels (r > 0.5), whereas such correlations were found for IL-8 and IL-10 in patients with SOFA scores ≥ 12 (n=9).

Table 2. Correlation of nucleosome levels with interleukin 6, 8 and 10

	LOD score (≥ 6) n=11		**SOFA score (≥ 12)** n=9	
	r	p	r	p
IL-6	0.573	0.060	0.750	0.0158
IL-8	0.646	0.029	0.817	0.004
IL-10	0.510	0.102	0.435	0.223

Abbreviations: LOD-score: Logistic organ dysfunction score, SOFA-score: Sepsis related organ failure assessment score, n: number of patients with a LOD score ≥ 6 or a SOFA score ≥ 12, IL: interleukin. r: Spearman rank correlation coefficient; p<0.05 was considered to be statistically significant.

Discussion

Despite considerable progress in basic support and new treatment options, MODS still contributes significantly to mortality of sepsis. MODS may hypothetically result from enhanced cellular apoptosis in the organs involved. Indeed, there is increasing evidence for a role of apoptosis in animal sepsis models and human sepsis (4,6,7). However, in spite of some indirect evidence (4,6,7), the involvement of apoptosis in human sepsis has not been established yet. We report here elevated plasma levels of nucleosomes, a specific and direct marker for apoptosis, in the majority of patients with sepsis or septic shock, and in a smaller proportion and at lower levels in patients with fever or SIRS, that were tested as controls. Thus, our data indicate enhanced apoptosis in patients with severe sepsis and septic shock.

Apoptosis of cells is detected by looking at specific cellular changes such as alterations of the phospholipid membranes, cell membrane permeability, condensation of cytoplasma and chromatin, and nuclear fragmentation. The latter results in a characteristic ladder pattern of DNA. However, assessment of these changes requires cells of the involved organs, which are not routinely available. As an alternative method to assess apoptosis of cells, plasma levels of the soluble form of Fas (sFas), which is the receptor for the TNF-like protein Fas-ligand, are often measured. Plasma levels of sFas are increased in patients with sepsis (6). However, elevated plasma levels of this truncated membrane protein per se do not conclusively point to enhanced apoptosis, since Fas may be cleaved off from cells by other processes, similarly as for example TNF-receptors. Even if the generation of sFas would be directly proportional to triggering by Fas-ligand, increased levels still do not necessarily reflect apoptosis. For example, the actual occurrence of apoptosis is influenced by a variety of intracellular pro- and anti-apoptotic regulatory proteins (18), which may result in uncoupling the apoptosis execution phase from the more upstream signal transduction processes, such as that induced by Fas. Hence, we took a different approach to assess apoptosis, i.e. we measured plasma levels of soluble nucleosomes. Nucleosomes consist of complexes of DNA fragments of 180 base pairs complexed to various histones, and are released by cells during the later stages of apoptosis. As they contain fragmented DNA, they constitute a direct parameter for apoptosis.

Circulating nucleosomes are undetectable in healthy subjects (Nieuwenhujize et al., manuscript submitted). Increased levels are expected to occur when the removal of apoptotic cells is impaired or when the number of apoptotic cells overrides the clearance mechanisms. Impaired nucleosome clearance likely explains their increased levels in some patients with systemic lupus erythematosus (10). We speculate that the increased levels found in patients with sepsis reflect increased formation with subsequent overloading of the clearance mechanisms.

We found no difference in nucleosome levels among patients with gram-positive or gram-negative infections. Also, patients with negative cultures had similar levels. Thus, cellular apoptosis in the patients occurred independently of the infecting organism, and hence is likely mediated by inflammatory mediators generated during sepsis. During sepsis, pro-inflammatory cytokines, such as TNF-α are released. TNF-α can interact with TNF-α p55 receptor, that shares homology with Fas-receptor (19). Either receptor can induce apoptosis via their intracellular death domains (19). TNF-α was only detectable in 15% of our patients on admission. However, IL-6, IL-8 and IL-10 responses are likely induced by this cytokine. Thus, the relationship between IL-6, IL-8 and IL-10 levels and nucleosome levels in the patients with high LOD- or SOFA-scores may point to TNF-α as a main inducer of apoptosis in sepsis. However, alternative mechanisms such as ischemia-reperfusion (20), in particular in the patients with shock, or complement activation products such as C5a (21) may have contributed as well.

Nucleosome levels showed a relationship to disease severity, as they were highest in severe sepsis or septic shock. Moreover, levels tended to be higher in non-survivors than in survivors. Interestingly, no clear correlation of nucleosome levels with clinical or laboratory parameters specific for a single organ were found. Hence, apoptosis in our patients does not seem to be restricted to a single organ. The lack of correlation with creatinine levels also excluded the possibility that the increased levels were due to impaired kidney function. Endothelial dysfunction likely plays a central role in sepsis, yet it is difficult to estimate in vivo (18,22). Dysfunction of endothelial cells may be due to apoptosis, for example induced by TNF-α. Other factors, like dispatchment of the endothelial cells from the extracellular matrix or low shear stress due to hypoperfusion may contribute to endothelial cell apoptosis as well (18). The positive correlations of nucleosomes with plasminogen activator inhibitor 1 (PAI-1) and tissue plasminogen activator (t-PA) levels at high LOD- and SOFA-scores (data not shown) suggest that the endothelium might be one of the potential sources of the nucleosomes measured in our patients (23). Apoptotic cells in their turn provide a strongly thrombogenic surface (18,24) and may enhance the procoagulatory state during sepsis. Thus, in addition to reduced organ perfusion, microvascular thrombosis could occur upon apoptosis of endothelial cells, thereby accentuating organ dysfunction.

In conclusion, we show for the first time elevated nucleosome levels in patients with sepsis. Our results suggest apoptosis, resulting from exposure of cells to excessive amounts of inflammatory mediators, to be pivotal in the pathogenesis of MODS.

References

1. Rangel-Frausto MS, Pittet D, Costigan M, et al: The natural history of the systemic inflammatory response syndrome (SIRS). *JAMA* 1995;273:117–123.
2. Bone RC: Toward a theory regarding the pathogenesis of the systemic inflammatory response syndrome: what we do and do not know about cytokine regulation. *Crit Care Med* 1996;24: 163–172.
3. Papathanassoglou EDE, Moynihan JA, Ackerman MH: Does programmed cell death (apoptosis) play a role in the development of multiple organ dysfunction in critically ill patients? A review and theoretical framework. *Crit Care Med* 2000;28:537–549.
4. Hotchkiss RS, Swanson PE, Cobb JP, et al: Apoptosis in lymphoid and parenchymal cells during sepsis: findings in normal and T- and B-cell-deficient mice. *Crit Care Med* 1997;25:1298–1307.
5. Leist M, Gantner F, Bohlinger I, et al: Tumor necrosis factor-induced hepatocyte apoptosis precedes liver failure in experimental murine shock models. *Am J Pathol* 1995;146:1220–1234.
6. Endo S, Inada K, Takakuwa T, et al: Nitrite/nitrate (NOx) and sFas antigen levels in patients with multiple organ failure. *Res Commun Mol Pathol Pharmacol* 1996;92:253–256.
7. Yamada Y, Endo S, Kasai T, et al: Nuclear matrix protein, tumor necrosis factor-alpha, and nitrite/nitrate levels in patients with multiple organ dysfunction syndrome. *Res Commun Mol Pathol Pharmacol* 1998;100:92–104.
8. Coutinho HB, Robalinho TI, Coutinho VB, et al: Intra-abdominal sepsis: an immunocytochemical study of the small intestine mucosa. *J Clin Pathol* 1997;50:294–298.
9. Earnshaw WC: Nuclear changes in apoptosis. *Curr Opin Cell Biol* 1995;7:337–343.
10. Amoura Z, Piette JC, Bach JF, et al: The key role of nucleosomes in lupus. *Arthritis Rheum* 1999;42:833–843.
11. Bossink AWJ, Groeneveld ABJ, Hack CE, et al: The clinical host response to microbial infection in medical patients with fever. *Chest* 1999;116:380–390.

12. Bone RC, Balk RA, Cerra FB, et al: Definitions for sepsis and organ failure and guidelines for the use of innovative therapies in sepsis. The ACCP/SCCM Consensus Conference Committee. American College of Chest Physicians/Society of Critical Care Medicine. *Chest* 1992;101:1644–1655.
13. Ziegler EJ, Fisher CF, Sprung CL, et al: Treatment of gram-negative bacteremia and septic shock with HA-1A human monoclonal antibody against endotoxin. A randomized, double-blind, placebo-controlled trial. The HA-1A sepsis study group. *N Engl J Med* 1991;324:429–436.
14. LeGall JR, Klar J, Lemeshow S, et al: The logistic organ dysfunction system. A new way to assess organ dysfunction in the intensive care unit. *JAMA* 1996;276:802–810.
15. Vincent JL, Moreno R, Takala J, et al: The SOFA (Sepsis-related organ failure assessment) score to describe organ dysfunction/failure. *Intensive Care Med* 1996;22:707–710.
16. Jansen PM, Van der Pouw Kraan TCTM, de Jong IW, et al: Release of interleukin-12 in experimental *Escherichia coli* septic shock in baboons: Relation to plasma levels of interleukin-10 and interferon-g. *Blood* 1996;87:5144–5151.
17. Helle M, Boeije L, de Groot E, et al: Sensitive ELISA for interleukin-6. Detection of IL-6 in biological fluids: synovial fluids and sera. *J Immunol Methods* 1991;138:47–56.
18. Mallat Z, Tedgui A: Apoptosis in the vasculature: mechanisms and functional importance. *Br J Pharmacol* 2000;130:947–962.
19. Bazzoni F, Beutler B: The tumor necrosis factor ligand and receptor families. *N Engl J Med* 1996;334:1717–1725.
20. Kohli V, Selzner M, Madden JF, et al: Endothelial cell and hepatocyte death occur by apoptosis after ischemia-reperfusion injury in the rat liver. *Transplantation* 1999;67:1099–1105.
21. Gua RF, Huber-Lang M, Wang X, et al: Protective effects of anti-C5a in sepsis-induced thymocyte apoptosis. *J Clin Invest* 2000;106:1271–1280.
22. Stefanec T: Endothelial apoptosis: could it have a role in the pathogenesis and treatment of disease. *Chest* 2000;117:841–854.
23. Vervloet MG, Thijs LG , Hack CE: Derangements of coagulation and fibrinolysis in critically ill patients with sepsis and septic shock. *Semin Thromb Hemost* 1998;24:33–44.
24. Bombeli T, Karsan A, Tait JF, et al: Apoptotic vascular endothelial cells become procoagulant. *Blood* 1997;89:2429–2442.

INFLAMMATION – INFECTION –SEPSIS

Finalists

Plasma Procalcitonin And C-Reactive Protein In Acute Septic Shock: Clinical And Biological Correlates

R. Claeys, S. Vinken, H. Spapen, K. ver Elst, L. Huyghens, F. K. Gorus

Academic Hospital Vrije Universiteit Brussel, Brussels, BELGIUM

Abstract

Introduction

Elevated procalcitonin (PCT) levels are markers of sepsis but their prognostic value and relation to other inflammatory parameters and calcium homeostasis remains controversial. We investigated whether in a cohort of patients with acute septic shock 1) PCT correlated with CRP, leucocyte count, ionized calcium (Ca^{2+}), clinical severity and survival; 2) diagnostic information provided by (changes in) PCT and CRP was similar.

Methods

Fifty-three patients with septic shock were consecutively diagnosed according to consensus guidelines. Blood was sampled at diagnosis, 24 and 48 h later and in a subgroup (n=23) after 120 h. PCT was measured with LUMItest (BRAHMS) and CRP with Vitros slides (Ortho). Ca^{2+} was calculated according to McLean-Hastings from calcium and protein levels on Vitros.

Results

In all 53 patients PCT and CRP were elevated (respectively > 0.5 ng/mL and > 10 mg/L) within 24 h after diagnosis. Non-survivors (n=25) were older ($p < 0.001$) and had higher APACHE II scores ($p = 0.02$) at diagnosis but did not differ in sepsis etiology, medical history, sex ratio, levels of PCT, CRP, and Ca^{2+} or WBC count at any time point. Using logistic regression, initial PCT levels correlated with CRP values ($p = 0.001$) and APACHE II score ($p < 0.05$), but not with age, gender, Ca^{2+} levels, survival or type of pathogen. Within 48 h, however, PCT levels decreased more frequently from baseline in survivors than in non-survivors (80% vs. 41%; $p < 0.05$). Likewise, CRP levels decreased more often in survivors (100% vs. 64%; $p < 0.05$) but only at 120 h.

Prevalence of decreasing plasma procalcitonin (PCT) and C-reactive protein (CRP) levels versus baseline values.

Time after admission	Characteristic	Survivors[a] n/n (%)	Non-survivors[a] n/n (%)	p
48 hours	Decreasing PCT[b]	20/25 (80)	10/21 (41)	0.047[c]
	Decreasing CRP	11/24 (55)	9/19 (45)	1.0[d]
120 hours	Decreasing PCT	12/12 (100)	9/11 (82)	0.22[d]
	Decreasing CRP[e]	12/12 (100)	7/11 (64)	0.037[d]

[a] missing data are due to insufficient serum sample or death of patients within 48 or 120 hours after onset of septic shock
[b] Odds ratio [95% confidence interval] for survival in patients with decreasing PCT levels during the first 48 hours after onset of septic shock: 4.4 [1.2–16.2]
[c] by Pearson Chi Square with Yates' correction
[d] by Fisher's Exact Test
e Odds ratio [95% confidence interval] for survival in patients with decreasing PCT levels during the first 120 hours after onset of septic shock: 15.0 [1.6–348.6]

Conclusions

PCT correlated with the severity of disease (APACHE II) and inflammation (CRP) but not with Ca^{2+} levels at diagnosis. Inaugural PCT or CRP levels *per se* poorly predicted outcome but decreasing levels were associated with a higher probability of survival. In this respect PCT was found to be an earlier marker than CRP.

Introduction

Sepsis and its sequelae are leading causes of mortality in ICU patients (1). Appropriate treatment of sepsis relies on early and correct diagnosis and contributes to a reduced morbidity and mortality. Conversely, more accurate diagnosis of sepsis will prevent overtreatment with broad spectrum antibiotics and vasoactive drugs. Sensitive and specific serum markers of the infectious origin and severity of systemic inflammation are needed to distinguish patients with systemic infection from those who appear septic but have no evidence of infection (2, 3). Though frequently used in routine, C-reactive protein (CRP) measurements appear far from ideal for this purpose since a marked rise in CRP has been described in the postoperative setting (4) and in non-infectious inflammatory conditions such as autoimmune and rheumatic diseases and myocardial infarction (5, 6). Furthermore, increased CRP levels are also found in minor or localized infections (7).

Procalcitonin (PCT) has recently been proposed as a potential specific marker of the systemic inflammatory response to infection (8, 9). Many clinical studies showed higher PCT levels in clinical bacteremia and sepsis than in systemic viral or localized bacterial infection (3, 8). PCT proved also valuable to discriminate infectious from highly inflammatory but non-infectious diseases, such as pancreatitis (10), cardiogenic shock (11), severe lupus (6), adrenal insufficiency (12) and acute transplant rejection (13).

However, the prognostic value of PCT in terms of survival in patients with sepsis and septic shock and the relation of PCT with other inflammatory parameters, such as CRP and white blood cell count (WBC), is still incompletely documented (14–16). Moreover, a possible role of PCT in the disturbed calcium homeostasis of sepsis remains a matter of debate (17–20). We therefore conducted a prospective study in a cohort of patients with acute septic shock, aiming [1] to determine the relation between plasma PCT levels, other markers of infection (CRP, WBC), serum ionized calcium (Ca^{2+}) levels, and patient outcome, [2] to compare the diagnostic and prognostic information provided by PCT and CRP levels.

Materials and Methods

Patients

The study was approved by the committee for Ethics in Human Research of the Academic Hospital of the Vrije Universiteit Brussels. Informed consent was obtained from the next of kin of each patient. Fifty-three patients (aged 18–93 years, median 66 years ; male-to-female ratio = 35:18) in whom septic shock was diagnosed within 4 hours of clinical onset, were consecutively enrolled between february 1996 and april 2000. Septic shock was defined according to consensus guidelines (21) as sepsis with hypotension resistant to fluid rescuscitation and evidence of organ hypoperfusion or dysfunction, namely: 1) hypotension: defined as systolic pressure under 90 mmHg or more than 40 mmHg reduced from baseline and 2) all of the following criteria: temperature > 38°C or < 36°, heart rate > 90/min, respiratory rate > 30/min or hyperventilation with arterial pCO2 < 32 mmHg, WBC > $12*10^9$/L or < $4*10^9$/L or more than 10% immature cells. Exclusion criteria comprised major thoracoabdominal (esophagectomy, Whipple's operation) or vascular surgery (abdominal or thoracic aneurysm resection) within 3 weeks before inclusion (associated with important post-operative increase of PCT levels as observed in ref 4), immunosuppressed state (treatment with corticosteroids, bone marrow or organ transplant recipients, leukopenia [WBC < $1*10^9$/L] or neutropenia [polymorphonuclear granulocyte count < 500/mL], hematological malignancy and AIDS), and a medical condition considered to be irreversible or lethal within 24 hours after admission. The analysis of the possible correlation between Ca^{2+} and PCT levels was performed before and after excluding patients with inherent disease-related hypocalcemia namely, patients with chronic renal failure (n = 5; retrieved from all patient's medical files and defined as having a plasma creatinine level above 250 µmol/L in stable conditions or being on hemodialysis or peritoneal dialysis);

patients with clinically established or suspected acute pancreatitis (n = 6; plasma lipase more than three times the upper reference limit) or patients with both conditions (n = 2).

All patients had indwelling radial (arterial line kit, Argon, Athens, TX, USA) and balloon-tipped pulmonary artery catheters (Edwards Swan-Ganz model 97-120-7F; Baxter Healthcare, Irvine, CA, USA) and, if required, were mechanically ventilated in volume- or pressure-controlled modes (Servo 900C ventilator; Siemens Elema, Solna, Sweden) under continuous analgesic sedation with midazolam and fentanyl. They received routine resuscitation therapy for septic shock, including fluid administration with crystalloids and colloids, dobutamine to maintain cardiac index 4L/min.m^2, and dopamine and/or norepinephrine to maintain mean arterial pressure > 65 mmHg. Following collection of blood and various culture material for microbiological analysis, all patients were given empirical broad-spectrum antibiotherapy which was later adjusted to culture results.

Clinical and Functional Investigations

The Acute Physiology And Chronic Health Evaluation (APACHE) II score was used to determine the initial severity of illness. A history of chronic renal failure was retrieved from the patients' medical files. Survival was defined as leaving the hospital alive and able to resume all previous daily activities.

Blood Sampling and Biochemical Assays

Blood samples were collected in K-EDTA (for WBC count) and lithium-heparin monovettes (Sarstedt, Essen, Belgium) at admission in the ICU and after 24 and 48 h and in a subgroup of 23 patients (enrolled between january 1998 and april 2000) after 120 h. Samples were immediately centrifuged at 3000 g for 10 minutes (Hettich Zentrifugen, Tuttlingen, Germany) and the plasma aliquoted and stored at –70°C. Total calcium and total protein concentrations were measured by colorimetric assays (Vitros analyser, Ortho Clinical Diagnostics, Rochester, NY, USA). Calculation of Ca^{2+} levels was based on the original Mc Lean-Hastings equation (22):

$$\text{ionized calcium} = \frac{6 \cdot \text{total calcium (g/dL)} - \dfrac{\text{total protein (g/dL)}}{3}}{\text{total protein (g/dL)} + 6}$$

Mc Lean-Hastings equation

Procalcitonin was measured by immunoluminometric assay (LUMItest PCT, BRAHMS Diagnostica GmbH, Berlin, Germany) and CRP by enzymatic immunoassay (Vitros CRP slide, Ortho Clinical Diagnostics). Cutoff values for PCT and CRP, were 0.5 mg/L and 10 mg/L, respectively.

Statistical Analysis

All statistical tests were performed with by the "SPSS for Windows 10.0" (SPSS Inc., Chicago, USA) statistical package for computers or with Epi Info version 6.0 (USD Inc., Stone Mountain, USA). Statistical differences between groups were assessed by Chi-square test, using Yates' correction or Fisher's exact test when appropriate, for categorical variables, and by the Mann-Whitney U test (unpaired values) or the Friedman or Wilcoxon test (paired values) for continuous variables. All tests were performed two-tailed and considered significant at $p < 0.05$ or, in case of k comparisons, when $p < 0.05/k$ (Bonferroni adjustment). Pearson correlation coefficients were calculated to estimate linear correlation between continuous variables. Multivariate analysis was performed by stepwise multiple linear regression after log-transformation of PCT levels. Normality of the residuals was verified by one-sample Kolmogorov-Smirnov test. Relative risk was calculated as an odds ratio (OR) using Woolf's formula with Haldane's modification [$OR = (2a+1)(2d+1)/(2b+1)(2c+1)$] when one element of the equation was zero.

RESULTS

Clinical, Demographic and Biological Baseline Characteristics of Patients with Septic Shock

Pneumonia was the most frequent underlying cause, followed by peritonitis and urosepsis (*table 1*). Most infections (31 of 53 or 58%) were caused by Gram-negative bacteria alone or in combination with other pathogens (*table 1*). In 44 patients (83%) one or more pathogenic infectious agents could be isolated or identified (*table 1*). In the remaining 9 patients no micro-organisms could be cultured, but in all of them the infectious focus was identified either clinically or at autopsy. All patients classified as non-survivors died in the hospital. There were no patients leaving the hospital alive with new disabilities. Non-survivors (n=25) were older than survivors (n=28) ($p < 0.001$) and tended to have higher APACHE II scores ($p < 0.02$) (*table 2*), but both groups did not differ in terms of underlying etiology of septic shock (*table 1*), sex-ratio, prevalence of acute pancreatitis and chronic renal failure nor in levels of PCT, CRP, WBC and Ca^{2+} (*table 2*).

Table 1. Origin of septic shock and microbiological findings

Type of infection	All (n=53)	Survivors (n=28)	Non survivors (n=25)
Pneumonia[a]	37	17	20
Peritonitis[b]	7	4	3
Urosepsis[c]	5	4	1
Catheter sepsis[c]	1	0	1
Meningitis[c]	1	1	0
Wound infection[d]	2	2	0
Type of pathogen			
Gram-negative	23	12	11
Gram-positive	8	5	3
Mixed (≥ 1 type of Gram-negative)	8	5	3
Anaerobe	1	1	0
Viral	2	1	1
Yeast	9	3	6

[a] The diagnosis of pneumonia was based on clinical and chest X-ray findings in all patients. Twenty-three patients grew pathogens on quantitative culturing of endobronchial secretions obtained by broncho-alveolar lavage or protected specimen brush. Thirteen patients had similar micro-organisms in bronchial aspirates and blood cultures, and in one patient pneumonia was confirmed at autopsy.

[b] Peritonitis was diagnosed peroperatively in all patients, two of them having also positive blood cultures.

[c] Blood cultures were positive in patients with catheter- or urosepsis and meningitis.

[d] The diagnosis of wound infection was made clinically.

Table 2. Demographic, clinical and biological characteristics at study inclusion

	All (n=53)	Survivors (n=28)	Non survivors (n=25)	*p*
Demographic				
Male-to-female ratio; n /n	35/18	20/8	15/10	0.56[b]
Age; years[a]	66 (52–73)	54 (40–68)	72 (65–78)	<0.001
Clinical				
APACHE II score[a]	24 (20–29)	22 (18–26)	27 (21–32)	0.02
Prevalence of acute pancreatitis or chronic renal failure; n/n(%)	13/53 (24)	6/28 (21)	7/25 (28)	0.81[b]
Biological				
PCT; μg/L[a]	5.9 (1.6–26.9)	4.3 (1.0–37.0)	10.3 (1.8–19.9)	0.44
CRP; mg/L[a]	199 (124–286)	197 (136–290)	212 (110–282)	0.78
WBC; X10^9/L[a]	14 (10–23)	14 (11–23)	13 (8–23)	0.53
Ca^{2+}; mg/dL[a]	4.0 (3.8–4.3)	4.0 (3.7–4.3)	4.0 (3.8–4.3)	0.82

[a] results are median (interquartile range)
[b] by Chi-square test with Yates' correction, all other p-values are calculated by Mann-Whitney U test
Threshold for statistical significance: p<0.05/8 or p<0.006 (Bonferroni adjustment)
APACHE = Acute Physiology And Chronic Health Evaluation; *PCT* = procalcitonin; *CRP* = C-reactive protein; *WBC* = white blood cell count; *Ca^{2+}* = ionized calcium

Clinical and Biological Correlates of Plasma PCT and CRP Levels at Baseline

At admission, univariate and multivariate analysis (*table 3*) disclosed a highly significant correlation of PCT levels with CRP concentration ($p = 0.001$) and with APACHE II score (univariate $p = 0.02$; multivariate $p = 0.05$) but not with Ca^{2+}, gender, age, survival and Gram-negative infection (*table 3*). Conversely CRP was only significantly correlated ($p = 0.001$) with PCT (*table 3*). Similar results were obtained when patients with acute pancreatitis or chronic renal failure (n = 13) were excluded from analysis (data not shown).

Table 3. Clinical and biological correlates of plasma procalcitonin (PCT) and C-reactive protein (CRP) at admission

	log PCT				CRP			
Variable analysis[b]	Univariate analysis[a]		Multivariate analysis[b]		Univariate analysis[a]		Multivariate analysis[b]	
	r[c]	p	ß[d]	p	r[c]	p	ß[d]	p
CRP[e]	0.45	0.001	0.44	0.001	–	–	–	–
log PCT[f]	–	–	–	–	0.45	0.001	0.45	0.001
WBC	−0.20	0.89	−0.23	0.12	0.04	0.39	0.14	0.31
Ionized Ca	−0.12	0.09	−0.13	0.40	−0.11	0.22	−0.02	0.86
APACHE II[e]	0.28	0.03	0.26	0.05	0.048	0.37	−0.08	0.55
Survival	na[g]	0.44	0.03	0.83	na[g]	0.45	0.05	0.73
Gender	na[g]	0.23	0.14	0.35	na[g]	0.41	−0.05	0.91
Age	na[g]	0.43	−0.09	0.57	na[g]	0.33	−0.05	0.71
Gram-neg. Infection	na[g]	0.70	0.08	0.59	na[g]	0.31	−0.18	0.19

[a] Pearson correlation for continuous variables after log-transformation of PCT levels and Mann-Whitney U test for categorical variables; threshold for significance p<0.05/8 or p<0.006 (Bonferroni adjustment)
[b] independent predictor ability of the variables studied by stepwise linear regression analysis after log-transformation of PCT levels
[c] Pearson correlation coefficient
[d] partial regression coefficient when all independent variables are expressed in standardized form
[e] nd
[f] variables selected in the stepwise linear regression for log PCT and CRP respectively ; for each of the other variables, the b-coefficient is that for the model in which the corresponding variable has been included in case of stepwise linear regression analysis
[g] not applicable

Evolution of Plasma PCT and CRP Levels during the Course of Septic Shock

All patients had elevated CRP concentrations within 48 hours after diagnosis. PCT levels exceeded cutoff values (> 0.5 μg/L) in 92% of patients at diagnosis, 100% after 24 h and 92% after 48 h. Survivors and non-survivors did not differ in prevalence of elevated PCT levels. Twenty-three patients were followed up to 120 h after admission. PCT levels were elevated during the first 48 h after admission in all of them and remained high in 78% at 120 hours (90% in non-survivors vs 67% in survivors; $p = 0.32$). CRP values in this subgroup invariably remained above cut-off.

Table 4. Changes in procalcitonin (PCT) concentrations at various time points versus baseline in 53 patients with acute septic shock[a]

Patients followed over 48 hours	Survivors	Non-survivors	P
PCT at admission; μg/L (n=53: 28 S, 25 NS)	4.3 (1.0; 37.0)	10.3 (1.8; 19.9)	0.436
PCT at 24 hours; μg/L (n=51: 28 S, 23 NS)[b]	4.8 (0.9; 35.1)	10.0 (3.5; 22.9)	0.272
change in PCT vs baseline; μg/L	-0.4 (-4.8; 0.3)	1.5 (-0.6; 5.6)	0.087
change in PCT vs baseline; %	-20 (-30; 30)	22 (-25; 85)	0.333
PCT at 48 hours; μg/L (n=47: 26 S, 23 NS)[b]	2.1 (0.8; 17.4)[c]	7.2 (3.2; 12.5)	0.294
change in PCT vs baseline; μg/L	-1.1 (-26.3; -0.1)	-1.1 (-26.3; -0.1)	0.262
change in PCT vs baseline; %	-55 (-63; -12)	5 (-47; 53)	0.312
Patients followed over 120 hours	**Survivors**	**Non-survivors**	**P**
PCT at admission; μg/L (n=53: 28 S, 25 NS)	5.7 (3.7; 61.9)	15.1 (1.7; 22.9)	0.747
PCT at 120 hours; μg/L (n=23: 12 S, 11 NS)[b]	0.9 (0.4; 4.7)[d]	1.7 (1.2; 2.4)[e]	0.622
change in PCT vs baseline; μg/L	-4.3 (-58.7; -1.8)	-9.7 (-18.2; -1.0)	0.275
change in PCT vs baseline; %	-87 (-92; -81)	-79 (-93; -38)	0.102

[a] all results are median (interquartile range); p-values are calculated by Mann-Whitney U test
[b] missing data are due to insufficient serum sample or death of patients within 24, 48 or 120 hours after onset of septic shock.
[c] significantly different from admission ($p = 0.003$) and values at 24 h ($p < 0.001$). Threshold for statistical difference: $p < 0.05/12$ or $p < 0.04$.
[d] significantly different from PCT at admission ($p = 0.002$). Threshold for statistical difference : $p < 0.05/4$ or $p < 0.012$.
[e] significantly different from PCT at admission ($p = 0.010$). Threshold for statistical difference : $p < 0.05/4$ or $p < 0.012$.
S = survivors, *NS* = non-survivors

Table 5. Changes in C-reactive protein (CRP) concentrations at various time points versus baseline in 53 patients with acute septic shock[a]

Patients followed over 24 hours	Survivors	Non-survivors	P
CRP at admission; mg/L (n=53: 28 S, 25 NS)	197 (136; 290)	212 (110; 282)	0.777
CRP at 24 hours; mg/L (n=51: 28 S, 23 NS)[b]	269 (197; 328)[c]	254 (153; 344)[d]	0.806
change in CRP vs baseline; mg/L	44 (−4; 70)	50 (−1; 100)	0.483
change in CRP vs baseline; %	20 (−1; 59)	28 (1; 71)	0.616
CPR at 48 hours; mg/L (n=47: 26 S, 23 NS)[b]	252 (192; 323)	228 (164; 250)	0.215
change in CRP vs baseline; mg/L	30 (−81; 98)	11 (−41; 82)	0.926
change in CRP vs baseline; %	12 (−34; 81)	5 (−33; 61)	0.944
Patients followed over 120 hours	**Survivors**	**Non-survivors**	**P**
CRP at admission; mg/L (n=53: 28 S, 25 NS)	226 (175; 331)	150 (70; 237)	0.134
CRP at 120 hours; mg/L (n=23: 12 S, 11 NS)[b]	89 (35; 140)[e]	142 (55; 182)	0.260
change in CRP vs baseline; mg/L	−162.3 (−209; −112)	−25 (−71; 18)	0.008
change in CRP vs baseline; %	−65 (−84; −81)	−25 (−54; 5)	0.011

[a] all results are median (interquartile range); p-values are calculated by Mann-Whitney U test

[b] missing data are due to insufficient serum sample or death of patients within 24, 48 or 120 hours after onset of septic shock.

[c] different from CRP at admission ($p = 0.052$). Threshold for statistical difference: $p < 0.05/12$ or $p < 0.04$.

[d] significantly different from CRP at admission ($p = 0.008$). Threshold for statistical difference: $p < 0.05/12$ or $p < 0.04$.

[e] significantly different from CRP at admission ($p = 0.002$). Threshold for statistical difference: $p < 0.05/4$ or $p < 0.012$.

S = survivors, *NS* = non-survivors

The PCT and CRP levels and their changes in time are presented in *table 4* and *table 5*. At each time point during follow-up PCT and CRP levels did not differ statistically between survivors and non-survivors (*table 4, table 5*) and no cut-off value discriminating survivors from non-survivors could be determined with receiver-operating chart (ROC) curve analysis (results not shown). However, only in survivors PCT values were overall lower at 48 h than at admission or at 24 h (p respectively 0.003 and <0.001). In patients followed over 120 h, a significant decrease in PCT levels vs. baseline values was observed both in survivors (p = 0.002) and in non-survivors (p = 0.01). Decreasing PCT levels within 48 h from baseline PCT occurred more often in survivors than in non-survivors (80% vs. 41%; $p < 0.05$) (*table 6*). The calculated odds ratio (95% confidence interval) for survival was 4.4 (1.2–16.2) in patients showing a decrease in PCT levels at 48 h. When only significant decreases in PCT were taken into account (i.e. a decrease of at least 3 times the coefficient of variation of the assay – which according to manufacturer's specifications corresponded to a 25% decrease in this study) the prevalence of decreasing PCT values also tended to be higher in survivors than in non-survivors (p = 0.08, not shown). At 120 h the frequency of decreasing PCT levels was similar in survivors and non-survivors (*table 5*).

Time after admission	Characteristic	Survivors[a] n/n (%)	Non-survivors[a] n/n (%)	p
48 hours	Decreasing PCT levels[b]	20/25 (80)	10/21 (41)	0.047[c]
	Decreasing CRP levels	11/24 (55)	9/19 (45)	1.0[d]
120 hours	Decreasing PCT levels	12/12 (100)	9/11 (82)	0.22[d]
	Decreasing CRP levels[e]	12/12 (100)	7/11 (64)	0.037[d]

[a] missing data are due to insufficient serum sample or death of patients within 48 or 120 hours after onset of septic shock
[b] Odds ratio [95% confidence interval] for survival in patients with decreasing PCT levels during the first 48 hours after onset of septic shock: 4.4 [1.2–16.2]
[c] by Pearson Chi Square with Yates' correction
[d] by Fisher's Exact Test
[e] Odds ratio [95% confidence interval] for survival in patients with decreasing PCT levels during the first 120 hours after onset of septic shock: 15.0 [1.6–348.6]

Twenty-four hours after admission, CRP levels tended to be higher than baseline levels both in non-survivors (p = 0.008) and in survivors (p = 0.053). An increase of CRP over baseline values during the first 24 h could not predict poor outcome in an individual patient (OR [95% CI]: 0.8 [0.2–2.8]; p = 0.964). CRP levels at 48 h did not differ from values at any previous time point in survivors and non-survivors (all p > 0.07), but at 120 h, they became significantly lower than baseline values in survivors (p = 0.002) but not in non-survivors (p = 0.374). Absolute and relative decrease in CRP at 120 h versus baseline values tended to be more distinct in survivors than in non-survivors (p-values respectively 0.008 and 0.011, significance lost after Bonferroni correction) (*table 5*). Survivors more frequently had decreasing CRP levels at 120 h than non-survivors (63% vs. 37%; p = 0.037), resulting in an odds ratio (95% CI) of 15.0 (1.6–348.6) (*table 6*). Based on manufacturer's specifications for assay imprecision and aforementioned criteria for significant changes in concentration with time, a significant decrease in CRP (by more than 25%) was observed after 120 hours in 91% of survivors vs. 46% of non-survivors ($p = 0.027$) (odds ratio [95% CI]: 13.2 [1.3–140.7]) for survival.

Discussion

The prognostic value of plasma PCT levels in predicting survival in adult septic shock is still controversial (15, 16). Previous studies were, however, performed in study groups of relatively small size (e.g. 24 surgical patients in ref 16) or of mixed composition (e.g. patients with sepsis or septic shock in ref 15). Therefore we conducted a prospective study in a larger cohort of 53 patients with acute septic shock.

In the present study, all patients had elevated PCT and CRP levels within 24 h after clinical diagnosis of septic shock. This is in agreement with previous observations in human sepsis (14) and septic shock (15, 16, 23). As was already suggested in septic patients (14) and/or in septic shock (15), baseline values of both markers *per se* failed to predict patient outcome because of a considerable overlap of ranges in survivors and non-survivors. Moreover, single PCT measurements during the first 5 days of treatment could not discriminate survivors from non-survivors. This is consistent with previous publications (14, 15) claiming that PCT levels only became significantly lower in survivors than in non-survivors during the second week of sepsis or septic shock; our results are at variance with another report (16) describing lower PCT levels in survivors than in non-survivors during the first 14 days after onset of septic shock in 24 surgical patients suffering predominantly from peritonitis and necrotizing pancreatitis.

PCT levels at admission were highly correlated with CRP and to a lesser extent with APACHE II score. CRP only correlated significantly with PCT. We and others (15) could not demonstrate a correlation between CRP concentrations and severity of disease or organ dysfunction scores. This further fosters the conviction that PCT better reflects the clinical severity of sepsis than CRP (3, 8, 15, 24). However, correlation coefficients between PCT and clinical scores remain low as shown by our and other studies (15) hereby invalidating the use of PCT as a surrogate for these scoring systems.

During the first 48 h after admission PCT levels overall significantly decreased only in surviving patients but not in non-survivors. The evolution in time of PCT levels provides better – though far from unequivocal – prognostic information with regard to patient outcome in septic shock than a single PCT measurement (14, 15). Decreasing plasma PCT levels during the first 48 h after admission slightly but significantly increase the probability of improved outcome.

With some exceptions (7), PCT has been described as an earlier and more specific marker of infection than CRP. PCT levels were reported to rise earlier after onset

(5, 24–26), and to decrease earlier during the course of sepsis than CRP. In contrast, the present study indicates that in septic shock patients CRP is a slightly more sensitive marker at diagnosis but tends to decrease later than PCT during follow-up. Significantly more survivors than non-survivors had decreased CRP levels at 120 hours.

In agreement with previous investigations (17, 21), hypocalcemia was a common finding in septic shock. Since a strong inverse correlation between PCT levels and total (19) or ionized (20) calcium was reported in both experimental and clinical studies on sepsis it was suggested that massive PCT release might mimic the biological activity of mature calcitonin. However, the present study found no correlation between ionized calcium levels and PCT values at admission, consistent with a direct role of PCT as independent pro-inflammatory mediator not affecting plasma calcitonin-like activity (27, 28).

In conclusion, baseline PCT and CRP levels are sensitive markers of acute septic shock but poorly predict outcome in terms of survival. Initial PCT levels were correlated with CRP levels and – unlike the latter – also to a lesser degree with APACHE II score, but not with Ca^{2+}. PCT decreased more frequently within 48 h after diagnosis in survivors than in non-survivors suggesting that the monitoring of PCT levels better predicts outcome than a single measurement. Similar findings were obtained for CRP but only at 120 h. Thus, compared to CRP, PCT levels are more related to the severity of the inaugural presentation of septic shock. Time-dependent changes in PCT concentration might provide an earlier indication on the chances of survival. The lack of correlation between ionized calcium and PCT levels, argues against a causal relationship between elevated PCT levels and hypocalcemia in septic shock unlikely.

Acknowledgements

The study was supported by the research and development funds from the departments of Clinical Chemistry and Intensive Care of the Academic Hospital of the Vrije Universiteit Brussel. We thank J.M. A-Tjak (BRAHMS Diagnostica, Berlin, Germany) for providing us with a luminometer and procalcitonin reagents and Prof. L. Kaufman (Dept. of Biostatistics, Vrije Universiteit Brussel) for statistical advice.

References

1. Rangel-Frausto MS, Pittet D, Costigan M, et al: The natural history of the systemic inflammatory response syndrome (SIRS). A prospective study. *JAMA* 1995; 273:117–123.
2. Natanson C, Hoffman WD, Suffredini AF, et al: Selected treatment strategies for septic shock based on proposed mechanisms of pathogenesis. *Ann Intern Med* 1994; 120: 771–783.
3. Karzai W, Oberhoffer M, Meier-Hellmann A, et al: Procalcitonin – a new indicator of the systemic response to severe infections. *Infection* 1997; 25: 329–334.

4. Meisner M, Tschaikowsky K, Hutzler A, et al: Postoperative plasma concentrations of procalcitonin after different types of surgery. *Intensive Care Med* 1998; 24: 680–684.
5. Karzai W, Meisner M, Reinhart K. New approaches to the diagnosis of sepsis. *Curr Opin Crit Care* 1999; 5: 357-362.
6. Eberhard OK, Haubitz M, Brunkhorst FM, et al: Usefulness of procalcitonin for differentiation between activity of systemic autoimmune disease (systemic lupus erythematosus/systemic antineutrophil cytoplasmic antibody-associated vasculitis) and invasive bacterial infection. *Arthritis Rheum* 1997; 40: 1250–1256.
7. Ugarte H, Silva E, Mercan D, et al: Procalcitonin used as a marker of infection in the intensive care unit. *Crit Care Med* 1999; 27: 498–504.
8. Assicot M, Gendrel D, Carsin H, et al: High serum procalcitonin concentrations in patients with sepsis and infection. *Lancet* 1993; 341: 515–518.
9. Whang KT, Steinwald PM, White JC, et al: Serum calcitonin precursors in sepsis and systemic inflammation. *J Clin Endocrinol Metab* 1998; 83: 3296–3301.
10. Rau B., Steinbach G, Gansauge F. The potential role of procalcitonin and interleukin 8 in the prediction of infected necrosis in acute pancreatitis. *Gut* 1997; 41: 832–840.
11. de Werra I, Jaccard C, Corradin SB, et al: Cytokines, nitrite/nitrate, soluble tumor necrosis factor receptors, and procalcitonin concentrations: comparisons in patients with septic shock, cardiogenic shock, and bacterial pneumonia. *Crit Care Med* 1997; 25: 607–613.
12. Hatherill M, Jones G, Lim E, et al: Procalcitonin aids diagnosis of adrenocortical failure. *Lancet* 1997; 350: 1749–1750.
13. Meisner M , Tchaikowsky K, Schmidt J. Indications for a new diagnostic parameter of severe bacterial infection and sepsis in transplantation, immunosuppression and cardiac assist devices. *Cardiovasc Engeneer* 1996; 1: 67–76.
14. Herrmann W, Ecker D , Quast S. Comparison of procalcitonin, sCD14 and interleukin-6 values in septic patients. *Clin Chem Lab Med* 2000; 38: 41–46.
15. Meisner M, Tchaikowsky K., Palmaers T. Comparison of procalcitonin and CRP plasma concentrations at different SOFA scores during the course of sepsis and MODS. *Curr Opin Crit Care* 1999; 3: 45–50.
16. Schröder J, Staubach KH, Zabel P; et al: Procalcitonin as a marker of severity in septic shock. *Langenbeck's Arch Surg* 1999; 384: 33–38.
17. Desai TK, Carlson RW, Geheb MA. Prevalence and clinical implications of hypocalcemia in acutely ill patients in a medical intensive care setting. *Am J Med* 1988; 84: 209–214.
18. Zaloga GP.Hypocalcemia in critically ill patients. *Crit Care Med* 1992; 20: 251–262.
19. Steinwald P, Whang K, Becker K. Elevated calcitonin precursor levels are related to mortality in an animal model of sepsis. *Curr Opin Crit Care* 1999; 3: 11–16.
20. Lind L, Carlstedt F, Rastad J, et al: Hypocalcemia and parathyroid hormone secretion in critically ill patients. *Crit Care Med* 2000; 28: 93–99.
21. American College of Chest Physicians/Society of Critical Care Medicine Consensus Conference: definitions for sepsis and organ failure and guidelines for the use of innovative therapies in sepsis. *Crit Care Med* 1992; 20: 864–874.
22. Weissman N, Pileggi VJ: Inorganic ions. In: Henry RJ, Cannon DC, Winkelman JW (Eds). Clinical Chemistry: Principles and Technics. Second Edition. Hagerstown (Maryland), Harper and Row Publishers Inc, 1974, p 664.
23. ver Elst K, Spapen H, Nguyen N, et al: Cardiac troponins I and T are biological markers of left ventricular dysfunction in septic shock. *Clin Chem* 2000; 46: 650–657.
24. Oberhoffer M., Karzai W., Meier-Hellmann A, et al. Sensitivity and specificity of various markers of inflammation for the prediction of tumor necrosis factor-a and interleukin-6 in patients with sepsis. *Crit. Care Med* 1999; 27: 1814–1818.
25. Monneret G, Labaune JM, Isaac C, et al: Procalcitonin and C-reactive protein levels in neonatal infections. *Acta Paediatr* 1997; 86: 209–212.
26. Brunkhorst FM, Heinz U, Forycki ZF. Kinetics of procalcitonin in iatrogenic sepsis. *Intensive Care Med* 1998; 24: 888–889.

27. Nylen ES, Whang KT, Snider RH Jr, et al: Mortality is increased by procalcitonin and decreased by an antiserum reactive to procalcitonin in experimental sepsis. *Crit Care Med* 1998; 26: 1001–1006.
28. Davis TM, Assicot M, Bohuon C, et al: Serum procalcitonin concentrations in acute malaria. *Trans R Soc Trop Med Hyg* 1994; 88: 670–671.

Macrophage Migration Inhibitory Factor And Hypothalamo-Pituitary-Adrenal Function During Critical Illness*

A. Beishuizen[1,3], L. J. Thijs[3], C. Haanen[2], I. N. Vermes[2]

Departments of Internal Medicine[1] and Clinical Chemistry[2], Medical Spectrum Twente, Hospital Group, Enschede, NETHERLANDS and Medical Intensive Care Unit[3], Free University Hospital, Amsterdam, NETHERLANDS

Abstract

Introduction

Macrophage migration inhibitory factor (MIF) is a multifunctional mediator with pituitary hormone, pro-inflammatory cytokine and catalytic enzyme activities[1]. MIF has the capacity to override the anti-inflammatory and immunosuppressive actions of glucocorticoids (GCs)[2]. MIF production is induced by low concentrations of GCs, but also by cytokines and stress activation. We evaluated the intriguing role of MIF in the complex network of immuno-neuroendocrine adaptation[3] during critical illness, by measuring blood levels of MIF and its relation with the HPA-axis, the acute phase response, cytokines, the severity of illness and ICU mortality.

Methods

In patients with septic shock (32), multitrauma (8) and hospitalised matched controls (40), we serially measured serum MIF, cortisol, DHEAS and plasma ACTH, TNF-α, IL-6 immunoreactivity for 14 days or until discharge/death. Also, serum levels of CRP, procalcitonin (PCT) and lipopolysaccharide-binding protein (LBP), all markers of the acute phase response, were determined. Statistical analysis was done using Kruskall-Wallis ANOVA, Spearman rank correlations and two-factor ANOVA.

Results

MIF was elevated (five-fold; $p<0.01$) in septic patients compared to trauma and control patients (see figure). There was distinct hypercortisolism on all days, with

* Paper originally published in the Journal of Clinical Endocrinology & Metabolism (86:2811–2816; 2001). Permission to republish in these proceedings was graciously granted by the Endocrine Society, Bethesda Maryland, USA.

a biphasic pattern of ACTH levels in both patient groups: high initially, paradoxically low from day 5. DHEAS was severely depleted in septic patients and to a lesser degree in trauma patients. MIF correlated strongly with serum cortisol (r_s=0.72; $p<0.01$). MIF also correlated significantly with IL-6, APACHE II and SOFA scores ($p<0.01$), but not with other variables (ACTH, DHEAS, CRP, PCT, LBP, TNF-α). MIF was higher in nonsurvivors and patients with ARDS ($p<0.01$).

Conclusions

MIF is significantly elevated in patients with septic shock, indicating that systemic inflammation leads to a prolonged stimulation of MIF release. MIF strongly correlates with cortisol, supporting its role as a contraregulator of GCs. MIF appears to have prognostic value considering its relation with mortality, the presence of ARDS and disease severity. Trauma patients show a discrepant pattern: normal MIF but increased cortisol levels, indicating a different regulation of GCs in these patients. The immuno-neuroendocrine interactions (possibly through IL-6) during immune-mediated inflammation (sepsis) are responsible for increased MIF release during septic shock and possibly explain this discrepancy. The stress-induced HPA activation appears to be less important as a trigger of MIF release, being present in both septic and trauma patients.

References

1. Swope MD, Lolis E. MIF: cytokine, hormone or enzyme? Rev Physiol Biochem Pharmacol 1999;139:1–32
2. Calandra T, Bernhagen J, Metz CN et al. MIF as a glucocorticoid-induced modulator of cytokine production. Nature 1995; 377:68–71
3. Beishuizen A. Immuno-neuro-endocrine adaptation in critical illness. Thesis. Vrije Universiteit 2001, Amsterdam

Introduction

Macrophage migration inhibitory factor (MIF) is a multifunctional mediator with pituitary hormone, macrophage-derived cytokine, and catalytic enzyme activities, which appear to be of pivotal importance to the regulation of the host immune and inflammatory response (1, 2). Based on animal studies, it has been shown that MIF displays a proinflammatory spectrum of actions that is most strikingly represented by its capacity to override the anti-inflammatory and immunosuppressive actions of glucocorticoids (GC) (3–6). MIF expression is biphasically regulated by GC, following a bell-shaped dose-response curve. At low physiological GC concentrations, MIF synthesis and release are induced, in contrast to any other cytokine, whereas at high GC concentrations its overriding capacity is diminished

(5, 7). There appears to be a dual role of MIF in optimizing inflammatory activity: being directly proinflammatory and indirectly inhibiting maximal antiinflammatory GC activity (1, 8). MIF release, the main source of which is the pituitary or monocytes/macrophages, is stimulated by inflammatory stimuli (microbial products and toxins), cytokines [tumor necrosis factor-a (TNF-α) and interferon-γ], and stressinduced activation of the hypothalamus-pituitary-adrenal (HPA) axis (4, 9–13).

During severe stress conditions, such as sepsis or trauma, activation of the HPA axis and hypercortisolism are present, whereas a discordant low ACTH level occurs in the chronic phase of critical illness (14). The antiinflammatory and immunosuppressive properties of GC are often beneficial in protecting the organism to mute its own inflammatory cascade (15), but to ensure host homeostasis the immunosuppressive effects of the HPA axis need to be counterregulated. Surprisingly, until recently no such system or no antagonizing mediator for GC was known. The rediscovery of MIF as a pituitary hormone/cytokine led to the awareness about MIF being a contraregulator to endogenous steroids within the host defense system (5, 16, 17).

Few data about the pathophysiological role of MIF in humans exist (17), although in animal models an important role is suggested in a variety of pathological conditions (18–25), such as endotoxic shock and the adult respiratory distress syndrome (ARDS) (4, 7, 9, 13, 26, 27). When coinjected into mice with lipopolysaccharide (LPS), MIF potentiates LPS lethality (9), whereas anti-MIF antibody offers full protection against lethal endotoxemia (4, 7, 9) and lethal bacterial peritonitis (27).

We investigated the intriguing role of MIF in the complex network of neuroendocrine adaptation during severe critical illness, such as severe trauma and septic shock, by measuring the time course of serum MIF levels in its relation to the HPA axis and to other cytokines, the severity of the disease, the occurrence of ARDS, and the final clinical outcome [intensive care unit (ICU) mortality].

Subjects and Methods

Study population

The study was performed in a total of 81 subjects. Approval for the study was obtained from our institutional human subjects research committee, and written informed consent from first degree relatives was mandatory. Forty consecutive patients admitted to the intensive care unit with septic shock or severe multiple trauma were included in the study within 6 h of admission.

Thirty-two patients had septic shock (12 females; mean age, 64 yr) as defined by clinical evidence of infection, temperature above 38.5 °C or below 35.6 °C, tachycardia (> 90/min), tachypnea (> 20/min), or necessity of mechanical ventilation. Shock was defined as a fall in systolic arterial blood pressure below 90 mm Hg, the need for vasopressors, together with signs of inadequate tissue perfusion (oliguria, mental alterations, lactic acidosis, coagulation abnormalities) (28). Eight patients (one female; mean age, 51 yr) were victims of multiple trauma of mechanical origin (injury severity score, > 20) (29).

Exclusion criteria were age below 18 yr, use of corticosteroids or other drugs affecting the HPA axis, unexplained hypo- or hyperkalemia, preexisting adrenal insufficiency or known abnormalities of the HPA axis, and multitrauma with head injury.

In both patient groups the severity of disease was scored according to APACHE II scores (30), multiorgan failure [sepsis-related organ failure assessment (SOFA) scores] (31), injury severity scores (29), the presence of ARDS, bacteriological findings, and clinical outcome (ICU mortality).

ARDS was defined as a condition involving impaired oxygenation (PaO_2/FiO_2, ≤ 200) regardless of the PEEP level, the detection of bilateral pulmonary infiltrates on the frontal chest radiograph, and a pulmonary capillary wedge pressure of 18 mm Hg or less or no clinical evidence of elevated left atrial pressure (32).

Control patients (18 females; mean age, 62 yr) were patients without acute medical illness admitted to the medical department for routine diagnosis and treatment. Written informed consent was obtained from all control patients. Patients with infectious diseases, autoimmune diseases, cancer, renal disease, and HPA abnormalities were excluded from this group.

Blood samples

Blood samples were drawn daily from arterial lines at 0600 h. Follow-up was performed for 14 days or until discharge from ICU or death. Blood was collected into plain tubes or into prechilled tubes containing ethylenediamine tetraacetate. Specimens were immediately centrifuged at 4 C and stored at –25 °C. Blood samples of the control subjects were collected by venipuncture between 0800–1000 h in the supine position after 30 min of rest. All hormone and cytokine measurements were performed in duplicate. Simultaneously, routine biochemistry (Roche, Basel, Switzerland) and hematology (HST 430, Sysmex Corp., Kobe, Japan) parameters were assessed.

Assays

Immunoreactive cortisol, ACTH, tumor necrosis factor-a (TNF-α), and interleukin-6 (IL-6) concentrations were measured with commercially available chemiluminescent enzyme immunoassays using the Immulite Automated Immunoassay System (Diagnostic Products, Los Angeles, CA). The cortisol assay is a solid phase chemiluminescent enzyme immunoassay that has an analytical sensitivity of 5 nmol/L and shows intra- and interassay coefficients of variation (CVs) below 7% measured at three levels.

Immunoreactive ACTH, TNF-α, IL-6, and LPS-binding protein (LBP) concentrations were measured with solid phase two-site chemiluminescent immunometric assays. The ACTH assay showed less than 0.001% cross-reactivity with ACTH-(1–18), ACTH-(1–24), ACTH-(22–39), and αMSH. The results were expressed as picomoles per L using ACTH-(1–39) as a standard. The assay has an analytical sensitivity of 0.2 pmol/L. The intra- and interassay CVs measured at three levels ranged from 3.1–8.2% and from 5.1–9.7%, respectively. The TNF-α assay showed no significant cross-reactivity to IL-2, -6, -8, or -10. The detection limit of the TNF-α assay was 2 ng/L, and the intra- and interassay CVs were less than 3% and less than 6%, respectively. The IL-6 assay showed nondetectable cross-reactivity to other ILs and 0.05% to TNF-α. The detection limit is 5 ng/L, and the intra- and interassay CVs measured at three levels were less than 6% and less than 10%, respectively. The LBP assay showed nondetectable cross-reactivity to IL-6, IL-8, TNF-α, and C-reactive protein (CRP). The analytical sensitivity was 0.2 mg/L, the interassay CVs measured at three levels were less than 10%, and the calibration range was up to 200 mg/L. Procalcitonin (PCT) concentrations were measured by an immunoluminometric assay using two antigen-specific monoclonal antibodies (LUMItest PCT, Brahms Diagnostica, Berlin, Germany). The minimal detected concentration with a maximal interassay CV was 0.3 μg/L. Immunoturbidimetric determination of CRP was made by an automated analyzer (Roche).

MIF serum levels were measured using a novel time-resolved fluorometry-based detection method (Delfia, Perkin-Elmer-Wallac, Inc., Gaithersburg, MD) (33). The results are expressed as micrograms per L using recombinant MIF as a standard (R&D Systems, Inc., Minneapolis, MN). The detection limit of the assay was 30 ng/L. The inter- and intraassay CVs varied from 1.2–3.1% and from 0.9–6.4%, respectively.

Statistical analysis

Values are expressed as the mean ± SD. All statistical analyses were performed using a statistical software package (version 9.0.1, SPSS, Inc., Chicago, IL). Qualitative values were analyzed using the χ^2 test. For data that were not normally distributed, the Mann-Whitney U test was used if only two groups were compared, and the Kruskal-Wallis one-way ANOVA test was used if more than two groups were compared. Serial data were analyzed using Friedman's repeated measures ANOVA on ranks, followed by Dunn's test for specific comparisons. The Spearman rank order correlation coefficient (r_s) was used to estimate the relation between MIF and the other variables. We used two-factor ANOVA to determine whether survivors and non-survivors as well as patients with ARDS and non-ARDS differed with respect to the MIF level and to calculate the interference between the presence or absence of survival and ARDS. The best cut-off for MIF was chosen using Youden's index, with calculation of sensitivity, specificity, positive predictive value (PPV), and negative predictive value (NPV). Then multiple logistic regression was used to test the predictive value of altered MIF concentrations and ARDS for outcome in patients with septic shock by calculating the odds ratios (OR) and its confidence limits (CI). For all statistical analysis, $P < 0.05$ was considered significant.

Table 1. Clinical and biochemical characteristic of the patient and control groups on admission to the intensive care unit

	Septic shock	Multiple trauma	Controls
Number	32	8	41
Age (yr)	64.2 ± 12.5[a]	51.7 ± 16.9[b]	62.1 ± 9.2
Gender (M/F)	20/12[a]	7/1[b]	23/18
Survivors	21[c, d]	8	41
Length ICU stay (days)	28 ± 8[c]	11 ± 4	
APACHE II	15.1 ± 5.5[a]	10.1 ± 2.1	
SOFA	8 ± 3.2[a]	4.2 ± 2.2	
ISS		24 ± 4	
Bacteriemia	20[c, d]	0	0
MIF (μg/L)	14.3 ± 4.5[c, d]	3.1 ± 1.7	2.5 ± 2.1
Cortisol (μmol/L)	1.21 ± 0.22[d]	1.08 ± 0.28[e]	0.31 ± 0.09
ACTH (pmol/L)	120.2 ± 28.2[d]	105 ± 36.5[e]	12.1 ± 4.2
TNFα (ng/L)	25.6 ± 10.7[c, d]	9.6 ± 2.1[b]	4.1 ± 2.3
IL-6 (ng/L)	1322 ± 388[c, d]	566 ± 266[e]	9.2 ± 4.2
CRP (mg/L)	171.2 ± 82[c, d]	39.2 ± 42.9	6.1 ± 3.2
LBP (mg/L)	41.7 ± 17.6[c, d]	9.1 ± 4.1	7.2 ± 4.2
PCT (μg/L)	33.2 ± 40.1[c, d]	1.34 ± 1.74	0.36 ± 0.33

Values shown are the mean ± SD. ICU, Intensive care unit; APACHE II, Acute Physiology and Chronic Health Evaluation; SOFA, sepsis-related organ failure assessment; ISS, injury severity score; MIF, macrophage inhibitory factor; TNFα, tumor necrosis factor-a, IL-6, interleukin-6, CRP, C-reactive protein; LBP, lipopoly-saccharide-binding protein; PCT, procalcitonin.

[a] $P < 0.05$, between septic shock and trauma.
[b] $P < 0.05$, between trauma and controls.
[c] $P < 0.01$, between septic shock and trauma.
[d] $P < 0.01$, between septic shock and controls.
[e] $P < 0.01$, between trauma and controls.

Results

Clinical and biochemical characteristics on admission of both patient and control groups are summarized in Table 1. Age, mortality, length of stay on ICU, and SOFA and APACHE II scores were higher ($P < 0.05$) in septic shock patients compared with multitrauma patients.

MIF was significantly ($P < 0.01$) elevated on day 1 in septic shock (14.3 ± 4.5 µg/L) as opposed to trauma patients (3.1 ± 1.7 µg/L) and controls (2.5 ± 2.1 µg/L). The time course of MIF as well as cortisol showed persistently elevated serum concentrations at all time points in septic shock independent of shock reversal (Figs. 1–3). ACTH levels displayed the characteristic biphasic pattern in both patient groups, with paradoxically low concentrations from day 5 (Figs. 2 and 3). In septic patients, we found on each individual day a strong positive correlation between MIF and cortisol levels (day 1: $r_s = 0.72$; $P < 0.01$; pooled data: $r_s = 0.77$; $P < 0.01$; Fig. 4). Also, on admission, a significant correlation was observed between MIF and IL-6 concentrations ($r_s = 0.40$; $P = 0.042$), APACHE scores ($r_s = 0.70$; $P < 0.01$), and SOFA scores ($r_s = 0.57$; $P < 0.05$). In both patient groups, no correlations in time were found between MIF and other variables (ACTH, TNF-α, CRP, PCT, and LBP).

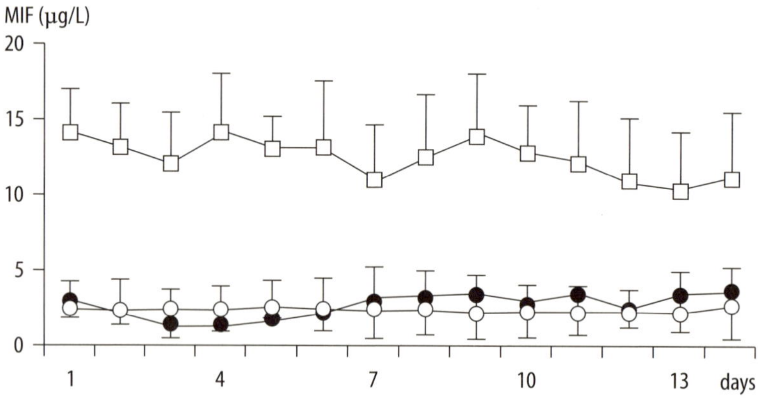

Fig. 1. Time course of serum MIF concentrations in patients with septic shock (□), multitrauma (●), and hospitalized matched controls (○).

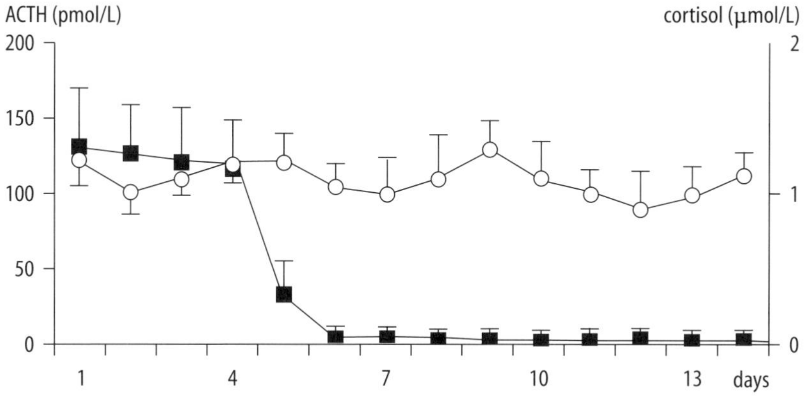

Fig. 2. Dissociation of serum cortisol (○) and plasma ACTH (■) concentrations in patients with septic shock.

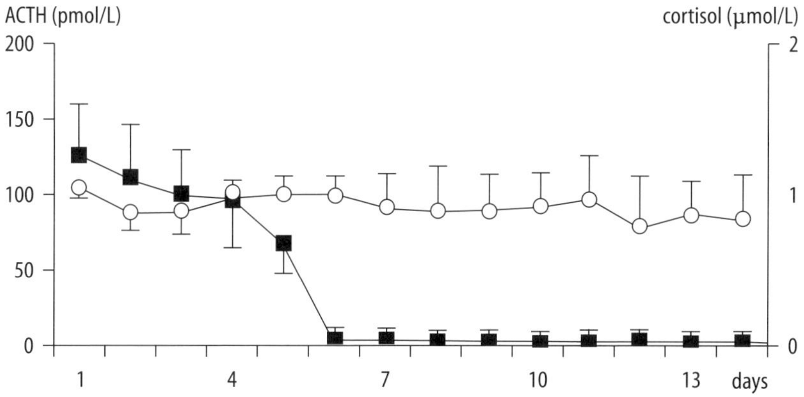

Fig. 3. Dissociation of serum cortisol (○) and plasma ACTH (■) concentrations in patients with multitrauma.

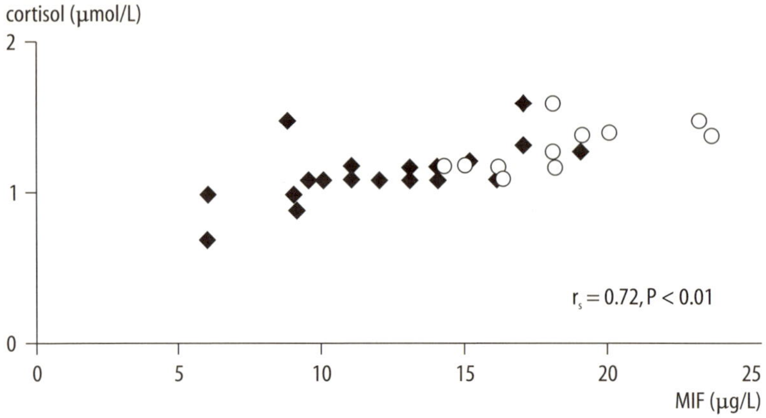

Fig. 4. Relation (Spearman rank correction coefficient r_s) between serum MIF and serum cortisol levels on admission in patients with sepsis. ◆, Survivors (n = 21); ○, nonsuvivors (n = 11).

A comparison between survivors and nonsurvivors and ARDS *vs.* non-ARDS in the septic shock group is shown in Table 2. Nonsurvivors showed higher MIF levels than survivors of septic shock (18.4 ± 4.8 and 10.2 ± 4.2 µg/L, respectively; $P < 0.01$). Patients with septic ARDS also had higher MIF levels than non-ARDS patients (19.4 ± 4.7 and 9.2 ± 4.2 µg/L, respectively). However, two-factor ANOVA showed a significant difference between MIF levels in survivors and nonsurvivors (F = 13.97; df = 1,28; $P = 0.001$), but no significant difference regarding ARDS (F = 2.67; df = 1,28; $P = 0.115$), and no significant interaction between survival or the presence of ARDS was observed (F = 0.65, df = 1,28; $P = 0.43$). Furthermore, we calculated the specificity, sensitivity, Youden's index, and predictive values for MIF levels on day 1 to determine a cut-off point that allows discrimination of patients with septic shock at risk for adverse outcome. A threshold of 14 µg/L showed a sensitivity of 82%, a specificity of 86%, a positive predictive value of 75%, and a negative predictive value of 90%. Multiple logistic regression analysis comparing increased MIF levels and ARDS in terms of relative risk for adverse outcome demonstrated that MIF was a better predictor of ICU mortality (MIF >14 µg/L: OR, 27; 95% CI, 3.8–191; $P = 0.001$ *vs.* ARDS: OR, 11.4; 95% CI, 1.74–76.9; $P = 0.01$).

Table 2. Comparison of clinical and laboratory data on admission between survivors vs. nonsurvivors and ARDD vs. non-ARDS in patients with septic shock (n = 32)

	Survivors	Nonsurvivors	Non-ARDS	ARDS
No.	21	11	24	8
Age (yr)	61 ± 11	67 ± 14	59 ± 13	64 ± 12
APACHE II	12 ± 5	18 ± 5[a]	11 ± 6	19 ± 4[a]
SOFA	6 ± 2	10 ± 4[b]	6 ± 3	11 ± 4[b]
Length ICU stay (days)	32 ± 7	24 ± 9[a]	24 ± 5	32 ± 11[a]
Bacteriemia	11	8[a]	12	7[a]
Gram-positive	2	2	3	1
Gram-negative	6[a]	9	6[a]	9
MIF (µg/L)	10.2 ± 4.2	18.4 ± 4.8[b]	9.2 ± 4.3	19.4 ± 4.7[a]
Cortisol (µmol/L)	1.15 ± 0.21	1.27 ± 0.23	1.11 ± 0.20	1.31 ± 0.24
ACTH (pmol/L)	115.1 ± 25.3	125.4 ± 31.1	111.5 ± 25.1	128.9 ± 31.3
TNFα (ng/L)	15.4 ± 9.9	35.8 ± 11.5[b]	17.3 ± 9.1	33.9 ± 12.3[b]
IL-6 (ng/L)	870 ± 377	1772 ± 399[b]	1130 ± 265	1514 ± 267[a]

Values are the mean ± SD. ARDS, Adult respiratory distress syndrome, APACHE II, Acute Physiology and Chronic Health Evaluation; SOFA, sepsis-related organ failure assessment; ICU, intensive care unit; MIF, macrophage inhibitory factor, TNFα, tumor necrosis factor-α; IL-6, interleukin-6.

[a] $P < 0.05$, difference between subgroups.

[b] $P < 0.05$, difference between subgroups.

In patients with multitrauma, MIF levels were not significantly elevated at any time point, in contrast to the high cortisol concentrations, and no correlation with cortisol or ACTH was present. A small subgroup of patients who developed infections (n = 3) also displayed normal MIF levels.

Discussion

HPA function plays a crucial role in metabolic and immunological homeostasis during critical illness (34). We (14) and others (35) showed that the HPA axis displays a biphasic pattern during the course of critical illness. The present data confirm high cortisol levels in these severely stressed patients together with the biphasic pattern of ACTH concentrations, showing paradoxically low concentrations in the chronic phase, indicating that cortisol release in this phase may be driven through an alternative (non-ACTH) pathway (14). Serum MIF, however, displayed significantly increased concentrations in critically ill septic patients. This release of MIF into the circulation indicates that the host also has the capacity to antagonize the systemic antiinflammatory properties of GC. However, it has been observed that MIF release follows a bell-shaped dose-response curve with respect to microbial toxins, and that its overriding capacity is diminished at high GC concentrations suggests the existence of counterregulatory mechanisms within the MIF/glucocorticoid system (1, 11).

We present the first data in humans directed upon the temporal course of MIF concentrations in severely ill patients suffering from multitrauma or septic shock. Patients with septic shock demonstrated increased MIF levels during acute and prolonged critical illness parallel to and strongly correlated with serum cortisol concentrations. Nonsurvivors, patients with positive blood cultures and ARDS, and the most severely ill patients showed the highest MIF (and cortisol) levels, suggesting that MIF might be an indicator of the severity of the septic shock. In animal experiments MIF acts to override GC-mediated inhibition of cytokine production (7). On the other hand, macrophage MIF is released upon stimulation with TNF-α, and at high levels (>100 μg/L) MIF induces TNF-α secretion by macrophages (27), augmenting each other in a proinflammatory loop (7). Our results showed high MIF and cytokine levels in the initial phase of septic shock, but a dissociation in the more chronic phase, when MIF levels were persistently high, whereas cytokine levels significantly decreased. We only observed a weak relation between serum IL-6 and MIF ($P = 0.042$) on admission, but no relation between TNF-α and MIF. IL-6 is a known activator of the HPA axis (36), but IL-6 is not known, in contrast to TNF-α or interferon-g, to induce MIF production (10).

Apparently both severe trauma and septic shock are conditions leading to activation of the HPA axis with a paradoxically low ACTH level during prolonged illness. However, the changes in MIF concentrations were distinctive; the persistently elevated levels of MIF in septic shock contrasted with the normal levels in multiple trauma. This fact suggests that the trigger of MIF release is not the stress-induced HPA activation, and the source of the high MIF concentration found in septic patients is not the pituitary. The bidirectional communication between the immune and neuroendocrine systems during the stress of inflammation could be the explanation for this discrepancy (37, 38). Possibly, endo- or exotoxins are more potent inducers of MIF release from the macrophages (4, 27) than the pituitary MIF release induced by hypothalamic activation during trauma. In fact, on admission we found significantly higher concentrations of IL-6, TNF-α, procalcitonin, and LBP in patients with septic shock than in patients with multiple trauma. Only IL-6 had a statistically significant relation, although weak, to serum MIF. No relation was present between MIF and procalcitonin, a promising marker and possible neuroendocrine mediator of sepsis (39, 40). We also examined the relation between MIF and LBP, a novel acute phase protein with possible protective effects against endotoxins (41–43). No relation was found between LPB and MIF levels on admission. Interestingly, LBP was strongly related to PCT, also an acute phase protein (data not shown). One can speculate that one of these substances could be responsible for the inflammation-induced MIF release in patients with septic shock.

Although MIF may function as a counterregulatory hormone for GC on inflammation and immune function in conditions of severe illness, its regulation must be different in view of the differences found in MIF levels between patients with septic shock and multiple trauma. In addition to its directly acting, proinflammatory functions, the secretion of MIF during immune-mediated inflammation suggests that there is a direct neurohumoral cytokine response to infection and tissue invasion. Its localization in central (pituitary) (9, 12) and peripheral (immune cells) (10, 44) sites is consistent with its pivotal physiological role within immune and endocrine defense systems (1, 17). Pituitary-derived MIF may serve to prime systemic immune responses once a localized inflammatory site fails to contain an invasive agent. Another explanation is that MIF acts as a central nervous systemderived stress signal to activate the immune system in anticipation of an impending invasive stimulus (9, 17). Accordingly, MIF may act in concert with ACTH and the adrenocortical axis to modulate systemic inflammatory responses (12). There is a sufficient molecular biological basis to suggest such an interplay between MIF and GC at the receptor/intracellular level (45–48). The antagonistic role of MIF regarding GC might be linked to its interaction with Jab1, by affecting $I_{\kappa}B_{\alpha}$ or by modulation of Jab1-steroid interactions (45).

In conclusion, we found markedly elevated serum MIF levels (5-fold) in septic shock compared with trauma and control patients. The prolonged stimulation of MIF release appears to be characteristic of septic shock, which supports the hypothesis that MIF might be a neuroendocrine modulator of systemic inflammation. In addition, nonsurvivors and more severely ill septic patients showed higher MIF levels at most time points. Also, we found markedly increased serum MIF levels in ARDS up to 14 days, which, in accordance with previously reported high local MIF levels in the lungs (49), suggests that the balance between MIF (proinflammatory) and cortisol (antiinflammatory) plays a role in the intensity of the inflammatory reaction. This might have important implications for GC treatment of sepsis or ARDS (8, 49–51). Both increased MIF levels and the presence of ARDS were independent predictors of adverse outcome.

GC are essential for survival during critical illness partly due to their potent antiinflammatory effects. However, GC also cause immunosuppression through GC receptor-mediated mechanisms. Prolonged, uncompensated elevation of GC receptor signaling would be maladaptive with regard to the immune system (46). GC might exert dual feedback effects at the level of the pituitary gland, inhibiting ACTH secretion while stimulating MIF secretion. High levels of MIF may be a crucial factor limiting the immunosuppressive effects of even high dose GC treatment for septic shock or late ARDS (52, 53). Anti-MIF therapy in combination with low dose GC may be considered an important treatment option for sepsis. In relative adrenal insufficiency, for which we are still searching for reliable diagnostic tests (54, 55), MIF might be the crucial factor in determining which patients will respond to GC therapy.

References

1. Metz CN, Bucala R. 1997 Role of macrophage migration inhibitory factor in the regulation of the immune response. Adv Immunol. 66:197–223.
2. Swope MD, Lolis E. 1999 Macrophage migration inhibitory factor: cytokine, hormone, or enzyme? Rev Physiol Biochem Pharmacol. 139:1–32.
3. Bernhagen J, Calandra T, Bucala R. 1994 The emerging role of MIF in septic shock and infection. Biotherapy. 8:123–127.
4. Calandra T, Spiegel LA, Metz CN, Bucala R. 1998 Macrophage migration inhibitory factor is a critical mediator of the activation of immune cells by exotoxins of Gram-positive bacteria. Proc Natl Acad Sci USA. 95:11383–11388.
5. Calandra T, Bucala R. 1997 Macrophage migration inhibitory factor (MIF): a glucocorticoid counter-regulator within the immune system. Crit Rev Immunol. 17:77–88.
6. Donnelly SC, Bucala R. 1997 Macrophage migration inhibitory factor: a regulator of glucocorticoid activity with a critical role in inflammatory disease. Mol Med Today. 3:502–507.
7. Calandra T, Bernhagen J, Metz CN, et al. 1995 MIF as a glucocorticoidinduced modulator of cytokine production. Nature. 377:68–71.
8. Morand EF, Leech M. 1999 Glucocorticoid regulation of inflammation: the plot thickens. Inflamm Res. 48:557–560.
9. Bernhagen J, Calandra T, Mitchell RA, et al. 1993 MIF is a pituitary-derived cytokine that potentiates lethal endotoxaemia. Nature. 365:756–759.
10. Calandra T, Bernhagen J, Mitchell RA, Bucala R. 1994 The macrophage is an important and previously unrecognized source of macrophage migration inhibitory factor. J Exp Med. 179:1895–1902.
11. Calandra T, Bucala R. 1995 Macrophage migration inhibitory factor: a counterregulator of glucocorticoid action and critical mediator of septic shock. J Inflamm. 47:39–51.
12. Nishino T, Bernhagen J, Shiiki H, Calandra T, Dohi K, Bucala R. 1995 Localization of macrophage migration inhibitory factor (MIF) to secretory granules within the corticotrophic and thyrotrophic cells of the pituitary gland. Mol Med. 1:781–788.
13. Bacher M, Meinhardt A, Lan HY, et al. 1997 Migration inhibitory factor expression in experimentally induced endotoxemia. Am J Pathol. 150:235–246.
14. Vermes I, Beishuizen A, Hampsink RM, Haanen C. 1995 Dissociation of plasma adrenocorticotropin and cortisol levels in critically ill patients: possible role of endothelin and atrial natriuretic hormone. J Clin Endocrinol Metab. 80:1238–1242.
15. Van den Berghe G, De Zegher F, Bouillon R. 1998 Acute and prolonged critical illness as different neuroendocrine paradigms. J Clin Endocrinol Metab.83:1827–1834.
16. Bucala R. 1996 MIF rediscovered: cytokine, pituitary hormone, and glucocorticoid-induced regulator of the immune response. FASEB J. 10:1607–1613.
17. Bernhagen J, Calandra T, Bucala R. 1998 Regulation of the immune response by macrophage migration inhibitory factor: biological and structural features. J Mol Med. 76:151–161.
18. Bernhagen J, Bacher M, Calandra T, et al. 1996 An essential role for macrophage migration inhibitory factor in the tuberculin delayed-type hypersensitivity reaction. J Exp Med. 183:277–282.
19. Lan HY, Bacher M, Yang N, et al. 1997 The pathogenic role of macrophage migration inhibitory factor in immunologically induced kidney disease in the rat. J Exp Med. 185:1455–1465.
20. Onodera S, Suzuki K, Matsuno T, Kaneda K, Takagi M, Nishihira J. 1997 Macrophage migration inhibitory factor induces phagocytosis of foreign particles by macrophages in autocrine and paracrine fashion. Immunology. 92:131–137.
21. Xu D, McSorley SJ, Tetley L, et al. 1998 Protective effect on *Leishmania major* infection of migration inhibitory factor, TNF-a, and IFN-gadministered orally via attenuated *Salmonella typhimurium*. J Immunol. 160:1285–1289.

22. Steinhoff M, Meinhardt A, Steinhoff A, Gemsa D, Bucala R, Bacher M. 1999 Evidence for a role of macrophage migration inhibitory factor in psoriatic skin disease. Br J Dermatol. 141:1061–1066.
23. Leech M, Metz C, Hall P, et al. 1999 Macrophage migration inhibitory factor in rheumatoid arthritis: evidence of proinflammatory function and regulation by glucocorticoids. Arthritis Rheum. 42:1601–1608.
24. Chesney J, Metz C, Bacher M, Peng T, Meinhardt A, Bucala R. 1999 An ssential role for macrophage migration inhibitory factor (MIF) in angiogenesis and the growth of a murine lymphoma. Mol Med. 5:181–191.
25. Martiney JA, Sherry B, Metz CN, et al. 2000 Macrophage migration inhibitory factor release by macrophages after ingestion of *Plasmodium chabaudi*-infected erythrocytes: possible role in the pathogenesis of malarial anemia. Infect Immun. 68:2259–2267.
26. Bozza M, Satoskar AR, Lin G, et al. 1999 Targeted disruption of migration inhibitory factor gene reveals its critical role in sepsis. J Exp Med. 189:341–346.
27. Calandra T, Echtenacher B, Roy DL, et al. 2000 Protection from septic shock by neutralization of macrophage migration inhibitory factor. Nat Med. 6:164–170.
28. Bone RC, Sibbald WJ, Sprung CL. 1992 The ACCP-SCCM consensus conference on sepsis and organ failure. Chest. 101:1481–3.
29. Baker SP, O'Neill B, Haddon Jr W, Long WB. 1974 The injury severity score: MIF AND HPA FUNCTION IN CRITICAL ILLNESS 2815 a method for describing patients with multiple injuries and evaluating emergency care. J Trauma. 14:187–196.
30. Knaus WA, Draper EA, Wagner DP, Zimmerman JE. 1985 APACHE II: a everity of disease classification system. Crit Care Med. 13:818–829.
31. Vincent JL, Moreno R, Takala J, et al. 1996 The SOFA (sepsis-related organ failure assessment) score to describe organ dysfunction/failure. Intensive Care Med. 22:707–710.
32. Bernard GR, Artigas A, Brigham KL, et al. 1994 The American-European Consensus Conference on ARDS. Definitions, mechanisms, relevant outcomes, and clinical trial coordination. Am J Respir Crit Care Med. 149:818–824.
33. Malmegrin KCR, Beishuizen A, Sluijs Veer van der GJ, Vermes I. 2000 Time-resolved fluorometric immunoassay of macrophage migration inhibitory factor. J Clin Ligand Assay. 20:74–80. 34. Beishuizen A, Vermes I, Haanen C. 2000 Hypotension, hypovolemia, and septic shock. In: Fink G, ed. Encyclopedia of stress, 1st Ed. New York: Academic Press; 460–468.
35. Naito Y, Fukata J, Tamai S, et al. 1991 Biphasic changes in hypothalamopituitary-adrenal function during the early recovery period after major abdominal surgery. J Clin Endocrinol Metab. 73:111–117.
36. Bethin KE, Vogt SK, Muglia LJ. 2000 Interleukin-6 is an essential, corticotropin-releasing hormone- independent stimulator of the adrenal axis during immune system activation. Proc Natl Acad Sci USA. 97:9317–9322.
37. Chrousos GP. 1995 The hypothalamic-pituitary-adrenal axis and immunemediated inflammation. N Engl J Med. 332:1351–1362.
38. Besedovsky HO, Del Rey A. 1996 Immune-neuro-endocrine interactions: facts and hypotheses. Endocr Rev. 17:64–102.
39. Braithwaite SS. 1998 Procalcitonin-marker, or mediator? Crit Care Med. 26:977–978.
40. Whang KT, Vath SD, Nylen ES, et al. 1999 Procalcitonin and proinflammatory cytokine in interactions in sepsis. Shock. 12:268–273.
41. Berczi I. 1998 Neurohormonal host defense in endotoxin shock. Ann NY Acad Sci. 840:787–802.
42. Lamping N, Dettmer R, SchroderNW,et al. 1998 LPS-binding protein protects mice from septic shock caused by LPS or Gram-negative bacteria. J Clin Invest. 101:2065–2071.
43. Opal SM, Scannon PJ, Vincent JL, et al. 1999 Relationship between plasma levels of lipopolysaccharide (LPS) and LPS- binding protein in patients with severe sepsis and septic shock. J Infect Dis. 180:1584–1589.

44. Bacher M, Metz CN, Calandra T, et al. 1996 An essential regulatory role for macrophage migration inhibitory factor in T-cell activation. Proc Natl Acad Sci USA. 93:7849–7854.
45. Kleemann R, Hausser A, Geiger G, et al. 2000 Intracellular action of the cytokine MIF to modulate AP-1 activity and the cell cycle through Jab1. Nature. 408:211–216.
46. Dorshkind K, Horseman ND. 2000 The roles of prolactin, growth hormone, insulin-like growth factor-1, and thyroid hormones in lymphocyte development and function: insights from genetic models of hormone and hormone receptor deficiency. Endocr Rev. 21:292–312.
47. Stocklin E, Wissler M, Gouilleux F, Groner B. 1996 Functional interactions between Stat5 and the glucocorticoid receptor. Nature. 383:726–728.
48. Daun JM, Cannon JG. 2000 Macrophage migration inhibitory factor antagonizes hydrocortisone-induced increases in cytosolic IkBa. Am J Physiol Regul Integr Comp Physiol. 279:R1043–R1049.
49. Donnelly SC, Haslett C, Reid PT, et al. 1997 Regulatory role for macrophage migration inhibitory factor in acute respiratory distress syndrome. Nat Med. 3:320–323.
50. Makita H, Nishimura M, Miyamoto K, et al. 1998 Effect of anti-macrophage migration inhibitory factor antibody on lipopolysaccharide-induced pulmonary neutrophil accumulation. Am J Respir Crit Care Med. 158:573–579.
51. Martin TR. 2000 MIF mediation of sepsis. Nat Med. 6:140–141.
52. Matot I, Sprung CL. 1998 Corticosteroids in septic shock: resurrection of the last rites? Crit Care Med. 26:627–630.
53. Meduri GU, Kanangat S. 1998 Glucocorticoid treatment of sepsis and acute respiratory distress syndrome: time for a critical reappraisal. Crit Care Med. 26:630–633.
54. Beishuizen A, Vermes I, Hylkema BS, Haanen C. 1999 Relative eosinophilia and functional adrenal insufficiency in critically ill patients. Lancet. 353:1675–1676.
55. Beishuizen A, Vermes I. 1999 Relative eosinophilia (Thorn test) as a bioassay to judge the clinical relevance of cortisol values during severe stress. J Clin Endocrinol Metab. 84:3400.

Early Identification Of High Risk Critically Ill Patients And Comparison With Acute Physiology Scores For Predicting Outcome

M. Manji, P. Gosling, and S. Brudney

Selly Oak Hospital, Birmingham, UK

Abstract

Introduction

Systemic inflammatory response syndrome (SIRS) leading to multiple organ failure (MOF) continues to be major problems following surgery and trauma, and accounts for up to 80% of deaths amongst critically ill patients (1). SIRS, characterised by a failure of inflammatory homeostasis, is the pathogenic mechanism linking these conditions. Experimental attempts to modulate mediators of the inflammatory pathway to attenuate this response have been disappointing(2). It is becoming clear that for such an approach to be successful, patients at risk must be identified very early in the course of their injury or insult (3).

A very early feature of inflammation is an increased capillary permeability to plasma proteins, which is amplified by the kidneys and can be monitored by measurement of low-level urine albumin excretion. This early identification of patients at risk of SIRS and MOF may allow effective intervention. This study examined microalbuminuria on admission to ICU with mortality, ICU stay, inflammatory response, organ function and was also compared with two (APACHE II, SAPS II) severity illness scoring systems.

Methods

Following Research Ethics Committee approval consecutive patients admitted to ICU were entered into the study. Urine albumin was measured by automated immunoturbidimetry and expressed as the albumin-creatinine ratio (ACR) in mg/mmol. APACHE II and SAPS II scores and their associated mortality probabilities were calculated based on physiological scores after 24 hours of admission. Statistical analysis was by Mann Whitney U test. The mortality predictive value of ACR, APACHE II and SAPS II were assessed using Receiver Operator Characteristic (ROC) curves. Association between ACR, physiological scores, ICU stay and markers of organ function and inflammation were made using Spearman rank correlation.

Results

140 patients were recruited. Results are shown below, median (95% CI)

$n = 140$	Survivors	Non-survivors	
Immediate ACR mg/mmol	4.2 (3.6–6.5)	17.8 (8.0–40.8)	$p < 0.001$
APACHE II score	21.0 (20.0–23.0)	25.5 (21.0–30.0)	$p < 0.05$
SAPS II score	44.5 (41.0–48.0)	63.8 (56.1–71.5)	$p < 0.001$

Surgical, trauma and burns patients (n = 92), but not medical patients (n = 48), showed significant association between ACR and ICU stay (rs = 0.32, p = 0.0021), highest serum C-reactive protein (rs = 0.40, p = 0.0002), serum creatinine (rs = 0.58, p = <0.0001) and bilirubin (rs = 0.36, p = 0.0009). The area under the mortality ROC curve for ACR, APACHE II and SAPS II mortality probabilities were 0.843 (p<0.0001), 0.793 (p=0.0004) and 0.770 (p = 0.0017) respectively.

Conclusion

ICU admission microalbuminuria was as good a predictor of outcome as APACHE II and SAPS II probabilities. ACR measurement shows promise as a simple predictor of risk of death at time of ICU admission in non-medical patients. This is in sharp contrast to APACHE II and SAPS II, which can only differentiate between survivors and non-survivors after 24 hours. Early identification by ACR of such at risk patients may allow immediate intervention or therapy aimed at modulating SIRS and subsequent MOF.

References

1. Baue AE, Durham R, Faist E Systemic inflammatory response syndrome (SIRS), multiple organ dysfunction syndrome (MODS), multiple organ failure (MOF): are we winning the battle? Shock 1998; 10: 79–89
2. Abraham E, Anzueto A, Gutierrez G et al Double-blind randomised controlled trial of monoclonal antibody to human tumour necrosis factor in treatment of septic shock. NORASEPT II Study Group Lancet 1998 ;351:929–33
3. Baue AE. Multiple organ failure, multiple organ dysfunction syndrome, and systemic inflammatory response syndrome: Why no magic bullets ? Arch Surg 1997;132:703–707

Introduction

Systemic inflammatory response syndrome (SIRS) leading to multiple organ failure (MOF) continues to be a major problem following surgery and trauma, and account for up to 80% of all ICU deaths, costing millions of pounds due to prolonged ICU bed occupancy(1). The pathogenetic mechanism which links these conditions is the systemic inflammatory response syndrome, defined as a failure of local control of the inflammatory response to injury or infection, allowing this process to over spill and damage organs remote from the site of injury (2). As the component parts of the integrated inflammatory response to injury and infection are identified, and their potential role in the development of SIRS studied, experimental attempts have been made to modulate key mediators in an attempt to attenuate this response (3–5). Since the release of key inflammatory mediators is extremely rapid, it is now becoming clear that for such an approach to be successful, patients at risk must be identified very early in the course of their injury or insult (6).

A very early feature of inflammation is increased capillary permeability to plasma proteins, which occurs within a few minutes of injury and usually returns to normal within 6 to 12 hours (7). Capillary leak is amplified by the kidney,[8] and can be monitored by measurement of low-level urine albumin excretion in the 20 to 200 mg/L range (microalbuminuria). Microalbuminuria reflects rapid changes in systemic capillary permeability and has been found to be predictive of outcome within a few hours of insult in a wide variety of acute conditions including trauma (9), surgery (10), ischaemia – reperfusion (11), acute pancreatitis (12), and meningitis (13). Failure of capillary permeability to return to normal, as assessed by microalbuminuria within 4 hours of surgery and 8 hours of trauma for example, has been shown to be a predictor of later organ failures (14). The suggestion has been made that it is timely to evaluate the predictive value of microalbuminiuria urine albumin excretion in patients requiring intensive care (15,16). A recent pilot study indicated that microalbuminuria, Six hours after admission to a general ICU, identified patients at high risk of developing sepsis syndrome and multiple organ failure (17). However no studies have yet been carried out to compare the clinical utility of microalbuminuria on admission to the ICU with severity of illness scoring procedures, mortality, length ICU stay and markers of inflammation and organ function in different clinical categories. This study aimed to compare microalbuminuria with mortality, acute physiological and chronic health evaluation score (APACHE) II, the simplified acute physiological score (SAP) II, and their derived mortality probabilities in patients admitted to a general ICU (18,19). Secondary aims were to compare microalbuminuria with duration of ICU stay and markers of inflammation and organ function.

Methods

Study Design

This was a prospective observational study. Microalbuminuria was assessed as the urine albumin creatinine ratio (ACR) on admission in unselected patients admitted to a general ICU. Admission ACR and APACHE II and SAP II scores (using data from the first 24 hours following admission) were compared with mortality on the unit and length of ICU stay for all patients and for subgroups of surgical, medical, trauma and burns patients.

Admission ACR was compared with laboratory markers of organ function (highest serum creatinine and bilirubin values during ICU stay) and markers of inflammation, (highest serum c-reactive protein and highest and lowest white blood cell count) during ICU stay.

Patients

Consecutive patients admitted to the ICU at Selly Oak Hospital, University Hospital Birmingham NHS Trust, were entered into the study. The ICU had 12 beds and received surgical, medical and trauma patients. There were no exclusion criteria other than anuria or failure to collect an admission urine sample. Patients admitted to the ICU or their relatives were informed of the study and invited to participate. The study was approved by the South Birmingham Local Research Ethics Committee.

Calculation of APACHE II and SAP II scores

APACHE II and SAPS scores were calculated from data collected during the 24 hours following ICU admission. APACHE II and SAP II scores were used to compute mortality probabilities.

Urine analysis

Ten mL of urine was collected from patients via a bladder catheter on admission to the ICU and frozen at −20 °C. Urine albumin was measured by automated immunoturbidimetry using rabbit antihuman albumin antibody (Dako™ High Wycombe, UK) with a limit of detection of 1.6 mg/L. Urine creatinine was measured after a 1:21 dilution by a modification of the Jaffe reaction on an ILab™ 900 automatic analyser. Results were expressed as the albumin-creatinine ratio (ACR) in mg/mmol. Values in a normal subjects are < 2.3 mg/mmol (< 20.3 mg/g) (14).

Statistical methods

Since ACR and ICU stay showed a skewed distribution, medians were compared using the Mann Whitney U test. APACHE II and SAP II scores were also compared using the Mann Whitney U test. The predictive value of ACR and mortality probabilities (derived from APACHE II and SAP II scores), were assessed by comparing the areas under Receiver Operator Characteristic (ROC) curves. Evaluation of any associations between ACR and physiological scores, ICU stay and markers of organ function and inflammation were made using the two tailed Spearman rank correlation procedure.

Results

Patients outcomes

Out of 140 patients studied, (92 male) mean (range) age 52.2 (16–92) years, 25 patients died in the ICU. Clinical categories are summarized in Table 1. Admission ACR, ICU stay and physiological scores after 24 hours for each clinical category are summarized in Table 2.

Table 1. Clinical categories of patients

Surgical		Trauma		Medical		Burns	
Vascular	30	Head Injury	8	Respiratory failure	12	Burns	6
Gastrointestinal	17	Multiple fractures	6	Asthma	7	Burns & smoke inhalation	4
Other	12	Abdominal injuries	3	Cardiac arrest	5	Scalds	1
		Stabbing	2	Sepsis	6		
		Trauma & head injuries	2	Cerebral bleed	4		
		Traumatic amputation	1	Pneumonia	3		
				Diabetes Mellitus	3		
				Guillian-Barre	2		
				Overdose	2		
				Meningitis	1		
				Pancreatitis	1		
				Hanging	1		
				Near drowning	1		
Total	59	Total	22	Total	48	Total	11

Table 2. Mortality and median (range) admission ACR, ICU stay and physiological scores after 24 hours by clinical category

Clinical category	n	Deaths	ACR mg/mmol creatinine: mg/g creatinine	ICU stay in hours	APACHE II score	SAP II score
All patients	140	25	6.1 (0.3–583.8): 53.9 (2.7–5160.8)	63.3 (8–1176)	22.0 (6–45)	49.5 (3–98)
Surgical	59	7	5.0 (0.3–180.5): 44.2 (2.7–1595.6)	48.0 (8–696)	23.0 (8–37)	40.0 (12–81)
Medical	48	14	8.9 (0.8–583.8): 78.6 (7.1–5160.8)	104.0 (16–1176)	23.0 (7–38)	57.5 (28–98)
Trauma	22	1	2.9 (0.4–40.5): 25.6 (3.5–358.0)	138.0 (9–575)	21.0 (8–29)	47.5 (16–67)
Burns	11	3	6.3 (0.3–134.0): 55.7 (2.7–118.5)	29.0 (12–912)	19.0 (6–45)	Not applicable

Comparison of admission urine ACR and physiological scores after 24 hours with mortality

For the whole group, urine ACR on admission was significantly higher in non-survivors, as were APACHE II and SAP scores (Figure 1 and Table 3). Urine ACR on admission and physiological scores after 24 hours for survivors and non-survivors, in subgroups of medical and non-medical patients (surgical, trauma, and burns) showed significant differences. For non-medical patients admission urine ACR, and 24 hour APACHE II and SAPS scores were again significantly higher in non-survivors (Figure 2 and Table 3). However for medical patients ACR and APACHE II scores showed no difference between survivors and non-survivors: only the mean SAP score was significantly higher in non-survivors (Figure 3 and Table 3).

Table 3. Comparison of median (95% CI) admission urine ACR and 24 hour physiological scores for survivors and non-survivors

Group	n	ACR mg/mmol creatinine: mg/g creatinine	APACHE II score	SAP score
All patients				
Non-survivors	25	17.8 (8.0–40.8): 157.4 (70.7–360.7)	25.5 (21.0–30.0)	63.8 (56.1–71.5)
Survivors	115	4.2 (3.6–6.5): 37.1 (31.8-57.5)	21.0 (20.0–23.0)	44.5 (41.0–48.0)
Difference in median (95% CI)		-8.20 (-3.8 to -18.8): -72.5 (-33.6 to -166.2)	-4.00 (-8.0 to -1.0)	-19.0 (-28.0 to -10.0)
Mann Whitney statistic	2129	1703.5	1730.5	
P	0.0002	0.0125	<0.00001	
Surgical, trauma and burns patients				
Non-survivors	11	23.7 (6.5–84.0): 209.5 (57.5–743.6)	28.0 (16.0–36.0)	66.0 (27.0–81.0)
Survivors	81	3.6 (2.6–4.6): 31.8 (23.0–40.7)	21.0 (19.0–23.0)	40.0 (31.0–47.0)
Difference in median (95% CI)		-15.50 (-23.0 to -5.4): -137.0 (-203.3 to -47.7)	-8.0 (-14.0 to -4.0)	-20.0 (-34.0 to -4.0)
Mann Whitney statistic	751	654.5	445.5	
P	0.0002	0.0017	0.0115	
Medical patients				
Non-survivors	14	10.7 (4.1–48.2): 94.5 (36.2–426.1)	23.4 (18.9–27.9)	61 (54.0–92.0)
Survivors	34	8.3 (5.7–10.8): 73.4 (50.4–95.5)	23.2 (20.2–26.3)	53.5 (45.0–63.0)
Difference in medians (95% CI)		-2.6 (-18.8 to 2.5): -23.0 (-166.2 to 22.1)	0.00 (-6.0 to 5.0)	-11.0 (-26.0 to -0.0)
Mann Whitney statistic	282	212	292	
P	0.3183	0.9201	0.0386	

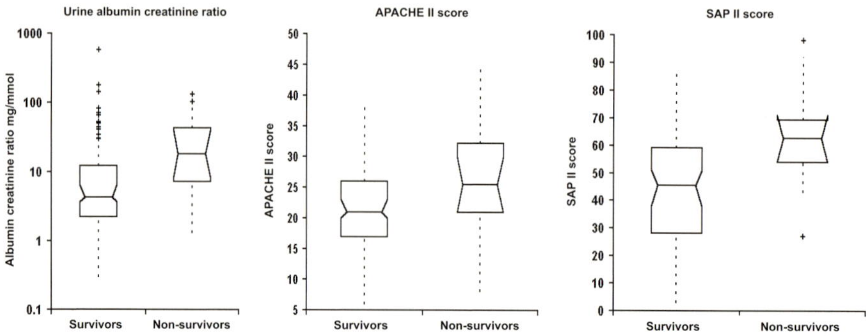

Figure 1. Comparison of admission ACR and 24 hour physiological scores for all patients. The boxes show the medians, the indents the 95% confidence intervals for the median, the upper and lower quartiles and the dotted line the 95% ranges. Values falling outside these limits are plotted individually.

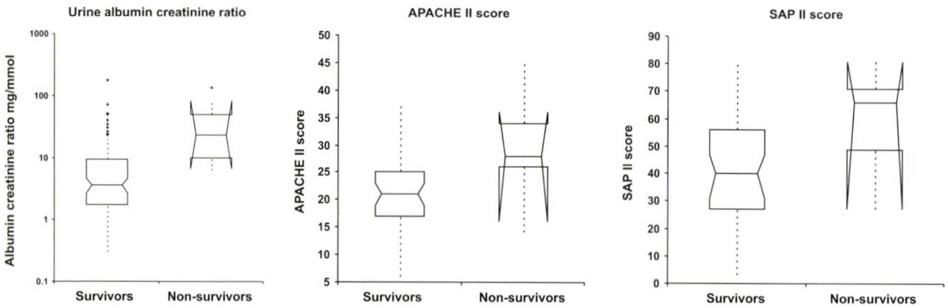

Figure 2. Comparison of admission urine ACR and 24 hour physiological scores for surviving and non-surviving surgical, trauma and burns patients. To convert ACR in mg/mmol creatinine to mg/g creatinine multiply by 8.84. (For details of box and whisker plot see legend to Figure 1)

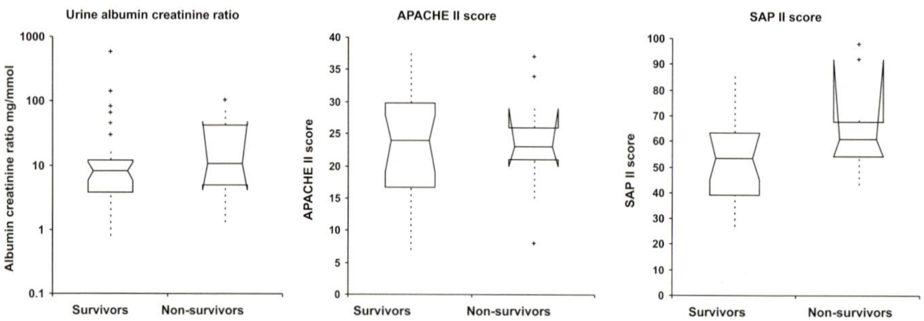

Figure 3. Comparison of admission urine ACR and 24 hour physiological scores for surviving and non-surviving medical patients. To convert ACR in mg/mmol creatinine to mg/g creatinine multiply by 8.84 . (For details of box and whisker plot see legend to Figure 1)

Comparison of ACR with APACHE II and SAPS II computed mortality probabilities

Comparison of the areas under ROC curves for all patients, showed that admission ACR and 24 hour APACHE II and SAP II mortality probabilities performed similarly in predicting death. (Table 4) Using a cut off for ACR on admission of 5.9 mg/mmol (52.2 mg/g) creatinine, the sensitivity for mortality was 84% with specificity of 56%.

For combined surgical, trauma and burns patients, ROC curves indicated that ACR on admission to ICU was equally as good a predictor of mortality, as mortality probabilities derived from APACHE II and SAP II scores determined 24 hours later. (Figure 4 and tables 4 and 5) Again using a cutoff of 5.9 mg/mmol (52.2 mg/g), ACR sensitivity for mortality was 100% with a specificity of 66%. The positive predictive value for death of an ACR of > 5.9 mg/mmol (52.2 mg/g) was 25%, with a negative predictive value of 100%.

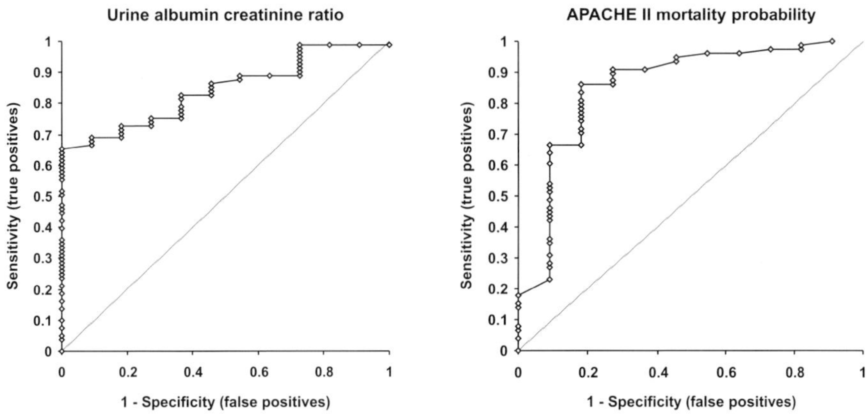

Figure 4. ROC curves for ACR on admission and APACHE II and SAPS II derived mortality probabilities for surgical, trauma and burns patients.

For the subgroup of 48 medical patients there was no association between mortality and ACR, however APACHE II and SAP II mortality probabilities were significant predictors of death (Table 4).

Comparison of admission urine ACR with physiological scores, ICU stay and markers of inflammation and organ function

For all patients, admission ACR was significantly associated with APACHE II and SAP II scores, length of ICU stay, highest serum c-reactive protein, creatinine, bilirubin and highest WBC (Table 5). These associations remained for combined surgical, trauma and burns patients with the exception of SAP II score: the association of ACR with highest WBC was of borderline significance (Table 5).

Table 4. Mortality ROC curve data

Clinical Group	Area under curve (95% CI)	p
All patients		
ACR	0.741 (0.638 to 0.843)	<0.0001
APACHE II mortality probability	0.796 (0.694 to 0.898)	<0.0001
SAP II mortality probability	0.786 (0.686 to 0.886)	<0.0001
Surgical, trauma and burns patients		
ACR	0.843 (0.753 to 0.933)	<0.0001
APACHE II mortality probability	0.793 (0.623 to 0.964)	0.0004
SAP II mortality probability	0.770 (0.590 to 0.950)	0.0017
Medical patients		
ACR	0.592 (0.405 to 0.780)	0.1664
APACHE II mortality probability	0.744 (0.588 to 0.900)	0.0011
SAP II mortality probability	0.731 (0.577 to 0.885)	0.0016

Table 5. Spearman Rank correlation data for admission ACR compared with physiological scores, ICU stay, inflammatory markers and highest serum creatinine and bilirubin.

	All Patients n=140		Non-medical patients n=94		Medical patients n=46	
ACR versus:	rs (95% CI)	p	rs (95% CI)	p	rs (95% CI)	p
APACHE II score	0.25 (0.08 to 0.40)	0.0039	0.25 (0.04 to 0.44)	0.0203	0.13 (−0.17 to 0.41)	0.3872
SAP score	0.26 (0.09 to 0.43)	0.0036	0.17 (−0.05 to 0.38)	0.1253	0.13 (−0.18 to 0.41)	0.4112
ICU stay	0.24 (0.08 to 0.39)	0.0036	0.32 (0.12 to 0.49)	0.0021	−0.06 (−0.34 to 0.23)	0.6721
Highest WBC	0.19 (0.03 to 0.35)	0.0218	0.20 (−0.01 to 0.391)	0.0581	0.12 (−0.17 to 0.39)	0.4040
Lowest WBC	−0.04 (−0.20 to 0.13)	0.6638	−0.12 (−0.32 to 0.09)	0.2592	0.14 (−0.15 to 0.41)	0.3297
Highest CRP	0.26 (0.09 to 0.41)	0.0038	0.40 (0.20 to 0.57)	0.0002	0.03 (−0.32 to 0.32)	0.8663
Highest creatinine	0.45 (0.30 to 0.57)	<0.0001	0.58 (0.43 to 0.71)	<0.0001	0.20 (−0.09 to 0.45)	0.1834
Highest bilirubin	0.24 (0.06 to 0.40)	0.0078	0.36 (0.15 to 0.54)	0.0009	0.22 (−0.08 to 0.49)	0.0052

For medical patients there was no significant association between ACR and APACHE II and SAP II scores, ICU stay or any of the inflammatory and organ function markers (Table 5).

There were no significant associations between admission ACR and ICU stay, physiological scores or markers of inflammation or organ function in trauma patients alone, with the exception of highest serum creatinine which showed a positive correlation with admission ACR (rs = 0.53 (95% CI 0.16 to 0.77) p = 0.0080). In the 11 burns patients, admission ACR was positively associated with ICU stay (rs 0.63 (95% CI) 0.05–0.89) p=0.037) highest serum CRP (rs=0.83 (95% CI) 0.47–0.96) p=0.0014), and highest serum bilirubin (rs=0.79 (95% CI) p = 0.0065) and negatively correlated with lowest white blood cell count (rs= –0.66 (95% CI) –0.90 to –0.10 p = 0.0269).

Discussion

Systemic inflammatory response syndrome and subsequent multiple organ failure carry a mortality of between 38 and 80% depending on the number of organs involved (1). Early identification of patients at risk of systemic inflammatory response syndrome is an essential precursor to development and evaluation of investigational interventions.

Illness severity scores were not intended for clinical decision making for an individual patient, but to compare disease severity between centers (20). However illness severity scoring data do provide a practical method for identifying patient populations suitable for new therapies and a method of evaluating new predictors of outcome. Two widely adopted systems to predict mortality are the acute physiological and chronic health evaluation (APACHE) II and the simplified acute physiological (SAP) II scores (16).

Attempts to use markers and mediators of the acute inflammatory response on admission to ICU following surgery or trauma, to identify patients at risk of later developing systemic inflammatory response syndrome, multiple organ failure and death, have had limited success. These include measurement of serum amyloid A, phospholipase A_2, neutrophil elastase, c-reactive protein (21), interleukin 6 and tumour necrosis factor alpha (22), soluble tumour nectosis factor receptors (23), and antioxidant status (24). Studies of tumor necrosis factor and interleukins 6 and 8 in patients with sepsis, revealed septic shock patients do not represent a homogeneous population in terms of their cytokine response (25).

In a study of 251 consecutive non-selected patients admitted to the ICU with septic shock, in which plasma tumor necrosis factor alpha, interleukin 6 and 8 concentrations were measured daily, APACHE II score remained the best predictor of mortality (26). The authors concluded that cytokine measurement is unlikely to have clinical application in the ICU setting, except possibly in specific subgroups of patients. In patients following severe trauma, endotoxin, tumor necrosis factor-alpha, interleukins 1 beta, 6, 8, and complement fragments C3a and C4a were not helpful in predicting the development of ARDS (27). Taniguchi et al (28) studied the time course of cytokine release following emergency department or ICU admission in order to identify patients suffering SIRS who are at risk of death. Failure of interleukin 6 to fall between days 0 and 4 and the interleukin 6 to 10 ratio were the best predictors of outcome. Recent studies assessing patients' haemodynanic status within a few hours of surgery either directly by ultrasonography (29), or indirectly by intramucosal tonometry (30), show promise but cannot easily be applied to every patient admitted to the ICU.

We have shown that a wide variety of acute inflammatory stimuli lead to transient microalbuminuria, which reflects changes in systemic microvascular permeability as part of the very early integrated acute inflammatory response. Normally microalbuminuria returns to normal levels within 4 to 12 hours of insult, but those patients with a sustained vascular leak, as evidenced by microalbuminuria, have a high risk of later organ dysfunction and death (15). It is likely than numerous inflammatory mediators and mechanisms are involved in the rapid dynamics of systemic vascular permeability, which may explain the similar response seen across a wide range of acute insults (15). The association of ACR on ICU admission with later maximum levels of both markers of inflammation and organ dysfunction is commensurate with this explanation. The speed and consistency of the microvascular response to acute injury, makes microalbuminuria an attractive candidate as an early marker of the severity of acute inflammation. A 1985 study of 50 ICU patients whose ACR was measured 6 hours after admission to a general ICU, showed it to be a good predictor of mortality and multiple system organ failure (18). The present study demonstrates that ACR on admission to ICU in combined surgical, trauma and burns patients, is as powerful a predictor of mortality as APACHE II and SAPS II predicted mortalities after 24 hours.

In previous studies of patients suffering severe blunt trauma, we showed that microalbuminuria was predictive of outcome 8 hours after admission (31,32). The lack of association of ACR with outcome or inflammation in trauma patients in this series may be due to the high proportion of head injury patients (10/22). Since ACR is related to the extent of tissue damage (33), even a catastrophic head injury will involve relatively small amounts of tissue and a limited inflammatory response. This effect was also seen with APACHE II scoring in a subset of non-operative head trauma patients in a recent multi-center study (34). Similarly the association between severity of inflammatory insult and capillary permeability may explain the close association between ACR on ICU admission and inflammatory and organ function markers in burns patients.

In medical patients, ACR does not predict mortality or correlate with ICU stay, APACHE II, SAP II scores or markers of inflammation and organ function. This may be because ACR is an early marker of the systemic inflammatory response to acute insult, which is likely to be variable in medical conditions such as chronic obstructive airways disease, asthma and diabetes. These patients may be predisposed to long ICU stays, not necessarily due to an acute insult, but because of pre-existing or chronic organ dysfunction and later nosocomial infection. This finding suggests that attempts to use markers of early inflammation as predictors of outcome in unselected critically ill medical patients may be unsuccessful.

For patients subjected to an acute insult such as surgery, measurement of ACR on ICU admission has the potential to discriminate between patients with a modest inflammatory response which resolves within a few hours, (predictive value for survival of 100%), from those patients suffering an exaggerated response (predictive value for death of 25%). ICU admission ACR may also provide a tool allowing early identification of patients with an exaggerated inflammatory response who would benefit from new therapeutic interventions aimed at attenuating the inflammatory process.

Acknowledgements

The authors wish to thank the nursing staff of the Selly Oak Hospital Critical Care Unit for their help in carrying out this study.

References

1. Baue AE, Durham R, Faist E Systemic inflammatory response syndrome (SIRS), multiple organ dysfunction syndrome (MODS), multiple organ failure (MOF): are we winning the battle? Shock 1998; 10: 79–89.
2. Davies MG, Hagen PO. 1997: Systemic inflammatory response syndrome Brit J Surg:84:920–35.
3. Jansen MJ, Hendriks T, Hermsen R, Van der Meer JW, Goris RJA A monoclonal antibody against tumour necrosis factor-alpha improves survival in experimental multiple organ dysfunction syndrome. Cytokine 1998; 11: 904–10.
4. Bone RC, Balk RA, Fein AM et al A second large controlled clinical study of E5, a monoclonal antibody to endotoxin: results of a prospective, multicenter, randomized, controlled trial. The E5 Sepsis Study Group. Crit Care Med 1995; 6: 994–1006.
5. Abraham E, Anzueto A, Gutierrez G et al Double-blind randomised controlled trial of monoclonal antibody to human tumour necrosis factor in treatment of septic shock. NORA-SEPT II Study Group Lancet 1998; 351: 929–33.
6. Baue AE. Multiple organ failure, multiple organ dysfunction syndrome, and systemic inflammatory response syndrome: Why no magic bullets ? Arch Surg 1997;132:703–707.
7. Fleck A, et al. Increased vascular permeability; a major cause of hypoalbuminaemia in disease and injury. Lancet 1985; I: 781–83.
8. Jensen JS, Borch-Johnsen K, Jensen G, Feldt-Rasmussen B. Microalbuminuria reflects a generalised transvascular albumin leakiness in clinically health subjects. Clin Sci 1995; 88: 629–33.
9. Pallister I, Gosling P, Alpar K, Bradley S. Prediction of post traumatic adult respiratory distress syndrome by albumin excretion rate eight hours after admission. J Trauma 1997; 42: 1056–61.
10. Smith CT, Gosling P, Sanghera K, Green MA, Paterson IS, Shearman CP. Microproteinuria predicts the severity of systemic effects of reperfusion injury following infra renal aortic aneurysm surgery. Ann Vasc Surg 1994; 8: 1–5.
11. Gosling P, Hughes EA, Reynolds TM, Fox JP. Microalbuminuria is an early response following acute myocardial infarction. Euro Heart J 1991; 12: 508–13.

12. Shearman CP, Gosling P, Walker KJ. Is low proteinuria an early predictor of severity of acute pancreatitis ? J Clin Path 1989; 42: 1132–5.
13. Roine I. Microalbuminuria: an index of severity in childhood menigitis. Pediatr Infect Dis J 1993; 12: 584–8.
14. Gosling P. Microalbuminuria: a marker of systemic disease. Br J Hosp Med 1995; 54: 285–90.
15. Gosling P, Bascom JU, Zikria BA. Systemic inflammatory response syndrome and magic bullets: finding the target and improving the aim. Arch Surg 1998; 133: 334.
16. Evans G, Greaves I. Microalbuminuria as a predictor of outcome: shows promise but large prospective trials are needed. Br Med J 1998; 318: 207–8.
17. MacKinnon KL, Molnar Z, Lowe D, Watson ID, Shearer E. Use of microalbuminuria as a predictor of outcome in critically ill patients. Br J Anaesth 2000; 84: 239–41.
18. Knaus WA, Draper EA, Wagner DP, Zimmerman JE. APACHE II: a severity of disease classification system. Crit Care Med 1985; 13: 818–29.
19. Lemeshow S, Teres D, Avrunin JS, Pastides H A comparison of methods to predict mortality of intensive care unit patients. Crit Care Med 1987; 8: 715–22.
20. Unertl K, Kottler BM. Prognostic scores in intensive care. Anaesthesist 1997; 46: 471–80.
21. Ensenauer R, Puttmann M, Quintel M, Kattermann R, Aufenanger J. Comparison of serum phospholipase A2, polymorphonuclear granulocyte elastase, C-reactive protein and serum amyloid A with APACHE II score in the prognosis of multiple injured pateinst. Clin Invest 1994; 72: 843–9.
22. Carlstedt F, Lind L, Linahl B. Proinflammatory cytokines, measured in a mixed population on arrival in the emergency department, are related to mortality and severity of diease. J Intern Med 1998; 242: 361–5.
23. Pilz G; Fraunberger P; Appel R; Kreuzer E; Werdan K; Walli A; Seidel D. Early prediction of outcome in score-identified, postcardiac surgical patients at high risk for sepsis, using soluble tumor necrosis factor receptor-p55 concentrations. Crit Care Med 1996; 24: 596–600.
24. Borrelli E; Roux-Lombard P; Grau GE; Girardin E; Ricou B; Dayer J; Suter PM. Plasma concentrations of cytokines, their soluble receptors, and antioxidant vitamins can predict the development of multiple organ failure in patients at risk. Crit Care Med, 1996; 24: 392–7.
25. Damas P; Canivet JL; de Groote D; Vrindts Y; Albert A; Franchimont P; Lamy M Sepsis and serum cytokine concentrations. Crit Care Med 1997; 25: 405–12.
26. Friedland JS; Porter JC; Daryanani S; Bland JM; Screaton NJ; Vesely MJ; Griffin GE; Bennett ED; Remick DG. Plasma proinflammatory cytokine concentrations, Acute Physiology and Chronic Health Evaluation (APACHE) III scores and survival in patients in an intensive care unit . Crit Care Med, 1996; 24: 1775–81.
27. Donnelly TJ; Meade P; Jagels M; Cryer HG; Law MM; Hugli TE; Shoemaker WC; Abraham E. Cytokine, complement, and endotoxin profiles associated with the development of the adult respiratory distress syndrome after severe injury. Crit Care Med, 1994; 22: 768–76.
28. Taniguchi T; Koido Y; Aiboshi J; Yamashita T; Suzaki S; Kurokawa A. Change in the ratio of interleukin-6 to interleukin-10 predicts a poor outcome in patients with systemic inflammatory response syndrome. Crit Care Med, 1999; 27: 1262–4.
29. Poeze M, Ramsay G, Greve JW, Singer M. Prediction of postoperative cardiac surgical morbidity and organ failure within 4 hours of intensive care unit admission using esophageal Doppler ultrasonography Crit Care Med 1999; 27: 1288–94.
30. Soong CV, Halliday MI, Hood JM, Powlands BJ, Barros D'Sa AA. The use of tonometry to predict mortality in patients undergoing abdominal aortic aneurysm repair. Eur J Endovasc Surg 1998; 15: 24–8.
31. Pallister I, Dent C. Wise CC, Alpar EK, Gosling P. Early post-traumatic acute respiratory distress syndrome and albumin excretion rate: a prospective evaluation of a 'point-of-care' predictive test. Injury 2001; 32: 177–81.
32. Pallister I, Alpar K, Bradley S. Prediction of posttraumatic adult respiratory distress syndrome by albumin excretion rate eight hours after admission. J Trauma 1997; 42: 1056–61.

33. Gosling P. Shearman CP, Gwynn BR, Simms MH, Bainbridge ET. Microproteinuria: response to operation Br Med J 1988; 296: 338–39.
34. Vassar MJ, Lewis FR Jr, Chambers JA, et al. Prediction of outcome in intensive care unit trauma patients: a multicenter study of Acute Physiology and Chronic Health Evaluation (APACHE), Trauma and Injury Severity Score (TRISS), and a 24-hour intensive care unit (ICU) point system. J Trauma 1999; 47: 324–9.

National Winners

4G/5G Promoter Polymorphism In The Plasminogen Activator Inhibitor-1 Gene In Children With Systemic Meningococcaemia

G. Geishofer[1], W. Zenz[1], B. Resch[3], S. Panzer[4], G. Endler[2], D. Häring[2], C. Mannhalter[2]

[1] Dept of Pediatrics, University of Graz, Austria
[2] Dept Laboratory Medicine, Division of Molecular Diagnostics, University of Vienna, Austria
[3] Dept of Neonatology, University of Graz, Austria
[4] Dept of Blood Transfusion, University of Vienna, Vienna, AUSTRIA

Abstract

Introduction

Fulminant meningococcaemia is a life-threatening disease with septic shock, disseminated intravascular coagulation (DIC), and hemorrhagic skin necrosis, and is associated with a high morbidity and mortality (1). Although meningococci are killed by antibiotics, the organisms or endotoxin trigger an intense host inflammatory response which leads to widespread endothelial injury with tissue damage and organ failure (2). The severity of meningococcal disease is related to the concentration of endotoxin, which in turn is related to higher concentrations of inflammatory mediators (3).

Patients with severe septic shock show the clinical syndrome of purpura fulminans, including severe disseminated intravascular coagulation with widespread micro- and macrovascular thrombosis, resulting in necrosis of the skin and infarctions of limbs and digits (4,5).

The pathophysiology of the coagulopathy in meningococcal sepsis seems to involve an imbalance of procoagulant and anticoagulant mechanisms. Concentrations of the anticoagulant proteins C, S and antithrombin III are low in plasma, the endothelial production of prostacyclin is impaired, thrombomodulin is down-regulated on the endothelial surface. while procoagulant molecules such as tissue factor are increased on monocytes (6). This leads to fibrin deposition and formation of microthrombi. Thrombosis also suggests impairment of fibrinolytic pathways, possibly due to endotoxin which has been shown to induce up-regulation of tissue plasminogen activator and plasminogen activator inhibitor 1 (PAI 1)(7).

PAI 1 is an acute-phase reactant, belonging to the serpin protease family and is synthesised and secreted by various cell types including endothelial cells, hepatocytes and platelets. It reacts with tissue and urinary plasminogen activators, as well as with protein C (8,9,10).

The concentration of PAI 1 is increased in inflammatory disease and high in plasma in patients with meningococcal sepsis. The highest concentration of PAI 1 is found in severe and fatal disease (11).

In the PAI 1 gene, a common, functional polymorphism, a single base-pair insertion (5G)/deletion (4G) polymorphism at nt (–675) has been identified, which is involved in the expression of the PAI 1 gene (12). In individuals with the 4G allele higher basal and inducible concentrations of PAI 1 have been found compared to those with the 5G allele.

In children of British and Dutch background, Hermans et al have shown, that carriers of the 4G/4G genotype, if they acquire meningococcal sepsis, produce higher concentrations of PAI 1, develop a more severe coagulopathy and have higher risk of lethal outcome (13).

These data have not yet been confirmed in other populations. Therefore, we designed a prospective multicenter study to investigate the association between the PAI-1 4G/4G genotype and mortality, amputation rate, and the extent of purpura in a middle European population.

Methods

Between January 2000 and August 2001 blood samples of 153 previously healthy children with invasive meningococcal infection were collected in more than 80 pediatric hospitals in Germany, Switzerland, Italy and Austria. The cohort includes 80 boys and 73 girls with a median age of 26 month (range 2–220 month).

The study was approved by the ethics committees of all participating hospitals and all parents gave written informed consent.

Meningococcal disease was diagnosed in patients by typical clinical symptoms such as fever, purpuric rash and meningitis, septicaemia or both or by isolation of meningococci from blood or cerebrospinal fluid, detection of meningococcal antigens, or positive PCR amplification of meningococcal genome in blood or cerebrospinal fluid.

Patients were classified to have meningococcal meningitis if they had evidence of meningism without the presence of shock or impaired peripheral perfusion, and meningococcal sepsis if they presented no evidence of meningism with features of shock or impaired peripheral perfusion (prolonged capillary refill time, tachycardia, raised base deficit, oliguria and impaired oxygenation)

Patients with both septicaemia and meningitis were classified as having combined disease.

Genomic DNA was isolated from whole blood by the Magna Pure DNA isolation kit (Roche Diagnostics). For determination of the 4G/5G polymorphism a newly developed mutagenic separated polymerase chain reaction assay (MS PCR) was used. MS PCR is a single tube PCR based technique relying on allele specific primers that differ in length by 8-10 base pairs (bp). Base mismatches at defined positions in the allele specific primers, introduced deliberately, minimize crossreactions of the PCR products generated from the two different alleles. Both alleles can be distinguished by length. In every sample, one or two different products are generated depending on the genotype.

Results

The genotype distribution in the patient group was in Hardy Weinberg equilibrium.

The prevalence of the homozygous 4G/4G genotype was higher in patients with amputations (40%) or death (37.5%) compared to survivors (24.3%). The difference was not statistically significant presumably due to the small number of patients with poor outcome, but the results correspond well with the data shown by Hermans et al.

Conclusions

Our data support an association between the homozygous 4G/4G genotype in the PAI 1 gene with mortality in children with meningococcal sepsis and are in good agreement with the results previously described by Hermans and Westendorp (12). Most likely we did not reach statistical significance because of the low number of patients with poor outcome, The association of the PAI-1 genotype with a poorer outcome in case of a meningococcal infection suggests, that increased levels of this inhibitor of fibrinolysis may play an important role in the pathogenesis of meningococcal septic shock

Previously, it has been demonstrated that individuals with the 4G/4G genotype produce six times more PAI-1 mRNA than carriers of the 5G/5G genotype in response to interleukin-1ß, a .macrophage product, which can be induced by tumor necrosis factor. Il-1ß stimulates the production of PAI activity in a concentration dependent way, with a maximal stimulation at 1 to 5 U/mL. The increase in PAI 1 and the impaired fibrinolysis can explain at least in part the extended of microvascular thromboses causally related with amputation of extremities or death in this disorder.

Measures to reduce the concentration of PAI 1 such as the administration of tissue plasminogen activator or activated protein C may be beneficial in patients with fulminant meningococcaemia. As has been demonstrated, treatment with activated protein C indeed significantly improves the outcome of sepsis.

In conclusion, genetic factors appear to play a role in septicemia. Further studies to confirm and extend our data are indicated.

References

1. Achtman M. Global epidemiology of menigococcal disease. In: Cartwright K, ed. Meningococcal disease. Chichester: John Wiley & Sons, 1995:159–77.
2. Nadel S, Levin M, Habibi P. Treatment of meningococcal disease in childhood. In Cartwright K, ed. Meningococcal disease. Chichester: John Wiley & Sons, 1995:207–43
3. Brandtzaeg P, Kierulf P, Gaustad P, et al. Plasma endotoxin as a predictor of multiple organ failure and death in systemic meningococcal disease. J Infect Dis 1989;159:195–204
4. Powars DR, Rogers ZR, Patch MJ, McGehee WG, Francis RB. Purpura fulminans in meningococcaemia, association with acquired deficiencies of proteins C and S. N Engl J Med 1987;317:571–72
5. Hazlezet JA, Risseeuw-Apple IM, Kornelisse RF, et al. Age-related differences in outcome and severity of DIC in children with septic shock and purpura. Thromb Haemost 1996;76:932–38
6. Moore KL, Andreoli SP, Esmon NL, Esmon CT, Bang NU. Endotoxin enhances tissue factor and suppresses thrombomodulin expression of human vascular endothelium in vitro. J Clin Invst 1987;79:124–30
7. Engebretsen LF, Kierulf OP, Brandtzaeg P. Extreme plasminogen activator and endotoxin values in patients with meningococcal disease. Thromb Res 1986;42:713–16
8. Pannekoek H, Veerman H, Lambers H, et al. Endothelial plasminogen activator inhibitor-1: a ew member of the serpin gene family.EMBO J 1986;5:2539–44
9. Ryan MP, Kutz SM, Higgins PJ. Complex regulation of plasminogen activator inhibitor type 1 (PAI 1) gene expression by serum and substrate adhesion. Biochem J 1996;314:1041–46
10. Zenz W, Muntean W, Gallistl S, Zobel G, Grubbauer HM. Recombinant tissue plasminogen activator (rt-PA) treatment in two infants with fulminant meningococcemia. Pediatrics 1995;96:144–8.
11. Kornelisse RF, Hazelzet JA, Savekoul HFJ, et al. The relationship between plasminogen activator inhibitor-1 and pro-inflammatory and counter-inflammatory mediators in children with meningococcal septic shock. J Infect Dis 1996;173:1148–56
12. Dawson SJ, Wiman B, Hamsten A, Green F, Humphfies S, Henney AM. The two allele sequences of a common polymorphism in the promoter of the plasminogen activator inhibitor-1 (PAI 1) gene respond differently to interleukin-1 in HepG2 cells. J Biol Chem 1993;268:10739–45
13. Hermans PWM, Hibbert ML, Booy R, Daramola O, Hazelzet JA, De Groot R, Levin M; et al. 4G/5G promotor polymorphism in the plasminogen-activator-inhibitor–1 gene and outcome of meningococcal disease. Lancet 1999;354:556–560

Quantification Of Viral Genomes In Immunocompromised Patients

B. Halima M.[1], Z. Arrouji[1], H. Dhaouadi[1], A. Slim[1], E. Ben Hassen[2], T. Ben Chaabane[3], S. Ben Redjeb[1]

[1] Microbiology laboratory, Charles Nicolle Hospital , Tunis, TUNISIA
[2] Laboratory of the National Center for Bone Marrow Transplantation, Tunis, TUNISIA
[3] Department of Infectious Diseases, La Rabta Hospital, Tunis, TUNISIA

Abstract

Introduction

The increasing prevalence of immunocompromised patients in Tunisia is due to the (1) immunosuppressive chemotherapy advances, (2) implantation of a national centre for bone marrow transplantation and (3) progressing number of HIV infected patients. Numerous infectious agents threaten these patients causing a significant morbidity often leading to hospitalisation in critical care settings. The monitoring of immunocompromised patients by molecular tools allows to reduce this morbidity and improve their life quality. In this study, we have routinely performed sequential quantification of CMV in transplant recipients since 1997 and the quantification of HIV-RNA in HIV infected patients since 2000.

Methods

Quantitation of CMV-DNA with the Hybrid Capture CMV DNA Assay

Three hundred and sixty eight blood specimens were obtained from the 128 patients (88 males and 40 females) from 1997 to 2000. These patients were essentially graft recipients (kidney : n = 48, bone marrow n = 61, liver : n = 1). Whole blood specimens were collected in EDTA tubes. After erythrocytes lysis, samples were centrifuged and the pellet resuspended in lysis buffer. Leukocytes were pelleted by centrifugation and stored at –20°C until testing. The assay, performed according to the manufacturer's instructions consists in : denaturation, probe mix addition, transfer to a capture tube and detection. Positive and negative calibrators are included in the test. Light emission was meseared in relative light units (RLU) and compared to the calibration curve.

Quantitation of plasmatic HIV-RNA with the Amplicor HIV-1 Monitor test

Whole blood specimens were collected in sterile EDTA tubes from 79 HIV-1 infected patients undergoing highly active anti-retroviral therapy (HAART) or naïve of treatment from November 2000 to April 2001. Plasma was collected after centrifugation and stored at –80°C until testing. The standard procedure of the assay was carried out as following : RNA extraction, reverse transcription followed by amplification and colorimetric detection. HIV-1 RNA was quantitated by utilizing the quantitation standard (QS) included in the test.

Results

CMV-DNA Results

Detection of CMV-DNA was positive in 31% of samples. Sequential samples were obtained from some patients. Quantitation results varied according to clinical findings and therapeutic efficacy. This monitoring has also revealed Ganciclovir-resistant viruses.

Plasmatic HIV-RNA Results

From November 2000 to June 2001, 79 consecutive samples were collected for viral load testing from HIV-1 infected patients. Among these patients, 37 (47%) were treated by triple antiretroviral regimen and 42 (53%) were naïve. Global results of HIV-1 RNA quantification are summarized in the table below:

	Undetectable viral load	**Viral load > 400 ARN-VIH copy/mL**
Total number of patients	18	61
Patients undergoing HAART	18	19
Naïve patients	0	42

Thus, only 49% (18/37) of patients receiving highly active antiretroviral therapy (HAART) had undetectable viral load. In addition, detectable viral load was more frequently associated with low CD4 cell counts and advanced stage of the disease.

Conclusions

Immunocompromised patients remain at significant risk of developing CMV infection and disease. In transplant recipients, the prevention of CMV pathologies is possible using laboratory monitoring for guiding prophylactic and preemptive strategies. The hybrid capture assay is reliable tool of detecting and quantifying CMV viremia. The improved sensitivity and the standardized format of the test allow inter-laboratory comparison.

Viral genomes quantification in transplantation settings enabled clinicians to initiate preemptive therapy of CMV infection and to evaluate its efficacy, reducing notably the morbidity and the mortality.

In HIV infected patients, the monitoring of plasmatic viral load allowed to indicate the prognosis of HIV infection and to determine when asymptomatic patients should be treated. It was also useful as a reference for subsequent monitoring of the virological response to therapy. The efficacy of antiretroviral therapy is measured by clinical improvement of the patient and by a favourable response of the biological markers (CD4 cell counts and plasma HIV-1 RNA). When these parameters were unfavourable, the therapeutic regimen could be changed. This monitoring delayed the occurrence of AIDS and opportunistic infectionsin our patients. Among treated patients, 51% had detectable viremia, suggesting anti-retroviral resistance. This will be documented by further studies.

Haptoglobin Polymorphism And Mortality In Patients With Tuberculosis

I. Kasvosve[1], Z. A. R. Gomo[1], E. Mvundura[1], V. M. Moyo[1], T. Saungweme[1], H. Khumalo[1], V. R. Gordeuk[2], J. R. Boelaert[3], J. R. Delanghe[4], D. De Bacquer[4], I. T. Gangaidzo [1]

[1] Departments of Medicine and Immunology , Medical School, The University of Zimbabwe, Harare, ZIMBABWE
[2] Department of Medicine, The George Washington University Medical Center, Washington, DC, USA
[3] Unit for Renal and Infectious Diseases, General Hospital St Jan, Brugge, BELGIUM
[4] Departments of Clinical Chemistry, and Public Health, University Hospital, Gent, BELGIUM

Abstract

Introduction

The three predominant phenotypes of haptoglobin are Hp 1-1, Hp 2-1 and Hp 2-2 and there are functional differences between the different haptoglobin phenotypes. As haptoglobin polymorphism has been considered a candidate genetic factor in the pathophysiology of tuberculosis, we conducted this study to determine whether susceptibility to clinical pulmonary tuberculosis is related to the haptoglobin phenotype; a second study question was whether the haptoglobin phenotype is predictive of outcome in patients treated for this condition.

Methods

Ninety-eight adults (44 females and 54 males) with sputum-positive pulmonary tuberculosis, were enrolled into the study at the time of diagnosis between June 1995 to June 1997. All study subjects were hospitalised at Nyadire Mission Hospital in the rural district of Mutoko, Zimbabwe. Subjects with symptoms suggestive of clinical pulmonary tuberculosis were referred for evaluation by a single team headed by the district tuberculosis officer. All cases of suspected or proven tuberculosis in the district are managed under the direction of this team.

A control group of 98 healthy adults from the same community and belonging to the same ethnic group (Shona), who were sex and age-matched to within five years was also recruited within 14 days of identifying a case. They were required to have a normal chest X-ray, absence of respiratory symptoms and a normal physical examination performed by a physician.

After collection, blood was kept chilled during transportation. Haematological tests were performed immediately on arrival at the laboratory the same day. Serum was stored at –80°C until biochemical analysis. The haptoglobin phenotype was determined by starch gel electrophoresis with haemoglobin-supplemented serum followed by peroxidase staining. Haptoglobin concentration was measured in 98 control subjects. Hepatitis B surface antigen marker for hepatitis B viral carriage was analyzed using enzyme immunoassay technique. A rapid test was used to test for antibodies to HIV-1 and -2.

Results

The haptoglobin (Hp) phenotype distributions did not differ significantly between the tuberculosis patients and controls (P = 0.5). During the 18 month follow-up period after starting tuberculosis treatment, 6/18 (33%) cases with Hp 2-2 phenotype died compared to 9/47 (19%) with Hp 2-1 and 3/31 (10%) with Hp 1-1. In a logistic regression model, the odds of dying were 6.1-fold greater with Hp 2-2 than with Hp 1-1 (95% CI of 1.04–35.1, P=0.04).

Conclusions

Our results suggest that there is equal susceptibility to clinical pulmonary tuberculosis disease amongst different haptoglobin phenotypes. Nonetheless tuberculosis patients with Hp 2-2 phenotype had a higher risk of mortality.

HYPOXIA – ISCHAEMIA

Finalist

Phospholipases A_2 Levels And Distribution In Bronchoalveolar Lavage Fluid Of Patients With Acute Respiratory Distress Syndrome (ARDS): Application Of A Fluorimetric Method

E. I. Kitsiouli[1], G. Nakos,[2] M. E. Lekka[1]

[1] Biochemistry Lab., Chemistry Dept., University of Ioannina, GREECE.
[2] Intensive Care Unit, University Hospital of Ioannina, GREECE

Keywords:
Phospholipase A_2, PAF-acetylhydrolase, ARDS, acute respiratory distress syndrome, bronchoalveolar lavage, NBD-lipids, fluorescence.

Abstract

Introduction

ARDS is a clinical syndrome with high mortality rates and is characterized by inflammatory injury and increased permeability alveolar-capillary edema.

Phospholipases (PLases) A_2 are the enzymes that hydrolyse phospholipids, the main constituents of lung surfactant. There are enzymic forms with preference to hydrolyze long or short fatty acyl chains at the *sn*-2 position and present different demand on calcium ions. PAF-acetylhydrolase (PAF-AcH) is a Ca^{2+}-independent enzyme which hydrolyses short fatty acyl chains. It is called PAF-AcH due to its capability to degrade platelet-activating factor (PAF), an inflammatory mediator.

PLases A_2 can affect adversely pulmonary function, directly by hydrolyzing surfactant phospholipids and increasing surface tension or indirectly with the production of inflammatory molecules and their metabolites or even by producing PAF. Experimental and clinical data indicate that PLase A_2 could be the major regulator in the development of inflammatory disorders which lead to the onset and evolution of ARDS (1). However, PAF-acetylhydrolase is considered as an anti-inflammatory enzyme since it hydrolyses and thus deactivates PAF.

The aim of this study was the fluorimetric determination of Ca^{2+}-dependent PLase A_2 and PAF-AcH activities and the investigation of the enzymes' distribution in surfactant fractions of BAL of ARDS patients.

Methods

Phospholipase A_2 and PAF-acetylhydrolase activities were measured using NBD-phosphatidylcholines as substrates (2). Surfactant was fractionated in its two different forms after ultracentrifugations of BAL. The lamellar bodies which are considered as "good" surfactant were obtained in the pellet of 30,000 g while the destroyed form of surfactant lamellar bodies were collected in 100,000 g pellet.

Results

Ca^{2+}-dependent phospholipase A_2 activity was detected in BAL of the patients (0.448±0.279 nmol C_{12}-NBD-FA/mg protein/h) while it was not detected in control group. PAF-acetylhydrolase activity levels were higher in BAL samples of ARDS patients (1.91±0.8 nmol C_6-NBD-FA /mg protein/h) than in control group (0.022±0.02 nmol/mg protein/h).

PLase A_2 total activity was distributed as 22.1, 2.6 and 75.3 % in the pellets of 30,000, 100,000 g and supernatant of 100,000 g, respectively. 51,1 % of PAF-AcH total activity was found in the pellet of 30,000 g, while 14 and 34,9 % in the pellet and supernatant of 100,000 g, respectively.

Conclusions

High levels of phospholipase A_2 indicate that this activity could play important role in pathogenesis and perpetuation of inflammation that characterize ARDS. PAF-AcH could contribute to the down-regulation of inflammation since it seems to correlate positively with the levels of inflammation. Different distribution for both total activities in surfactant fractions indicate that lung PAF-AcH presents lipophilic properties while alveolar PLase A_2 is a water soluble enzyme. The study of the levels for both enzymes could give information about the severity and evolution of the disease. It could also be a useful tool for the evaluation of a therapeutic approach.

References

1 Touqui L, Arbibe L. A role for phospholipase A_2 in ARDS pathogenesis. Mol Med Today 1999; 5:244–9.

2 Kitsiouli EI, Nakos G, Lekka ME. Differential determination of phospholipase A_2 and PAF-acetylhydrolase in biological fluids using fluorescent substrates. J Lipid Res 1999; 40:2346–56.

Abbreviations

ARDS:	Acute Respiratory Distress Syndrome;
BSA:	Bovine Serum Albumin;
C_6-NBD-PC:	1-palmitoyl-2-[6-[(7-nitro-2-1,3-benzoxadiazol-4-yl)amino] hexanoyl]-*sn*-glycero-3-phosphocholine;
C_{12}-NBD-PC:	1-palmitoyl-2-[12-[(7-nitro-2-1,3-benzoxadiazol-4-yl)amino] dodecanoyl]-*sn*-glycero-3-phosphocholine;
C_6-NBD-FA:	6-[(7-nitro-2-1,3-benzoxadiazol-4-yl)amino] hexanoic acid;
C_{12}-NBD-FA:	12-[(7-nitro-2-1,3-benzoxadiazol-4-yl)amino] dodecanoic acid;
LSA:	large surfactant aggregates;
SSA:	small surfactant aggregates;
VSSA:	very small surfactant aggregates;
DPPC:	dipalmitoyl-phosphatidylcholine;
BAL(F):	bronchoalveolar lavage (fluid);
PLase A_2:	phospholipase A_2;
AcH:	acetylhydrolase;
PAF:	Platelet-activating factor, 1-*O*-alkyl-2-acetyl-*sn*-glycero-3-phosphocholine;
PC:	1,2-diacyl-*sn*-glycero-3-phosphocholine;
EDTA:	ethylenediamino-tetraacetic acid;
FA:	Fatty Acid;
TLC:	thin layer chromatography;

Introduction

Phospholipases A_2 are a broad family of enzymes, which hydrolyze the ester bond at the *sn*-2 position of glycerophospholipids. Mammalian phospholipases A_2 are classified mainly on the basis of aminoacid sequence, origin (secretory or cytosolic forms), calcium requirements and substrate specificity (1,2). Ca^{2+}-dependent phospholipases A_2 give rise to the formation of potent lipid mediators such as arachidonic acid and eicosanoids, lyso-phospholipids and platelet-activating factor (PAF) (3,4). Platelet-activating factor acetylhydrolase (PAF-AcH) is a Ca^{2+}-independent phospholipase A_2 that cleaves the acetyl-group from PAF, as well as short, oxidatively-fragmented acyl groups from phospholipids, contributing to their deactivation (5,6).

Phospholipase A_2 can affect pulmonary function, directly by hydrolyzing lung surfactant phospholipids and increasing surface tension (7,8) or indirectly with the production of biologically-active molecules. The implication of phospholipase A_2 and PAF-acetylhydrolase in various lung diseases has been pointed out by a number of research groups: High phospholipase A_2 concentrations have been found either at the sites of inflammation or in circulation of patients with ARDS. Increased levels of PLase A_2, and/or PAF were detected in the acute respiratory distress syndrome (ARDS) (9–11), multiple organ dysfunction syndrome (12,13) and in septic shock (14). Positive correlation between phospholipase A_2 levels and the severity of lung injury was also observed. High levels of PAF-acetylhydrolase activity were detected in bronchoalveolar lavage fluid from patients with pulmonary inosis (15), ARDS (16) and pulmonary embolism (17). PAF-AcH was also detected in bronchoalveolar lavage (BAL) of patients with hydrostatic pulmonary edema (18) and it was inversely correlated with PAF levels.

In recent years, there has been an increased appreciation that biochemical inflammatory mediators, like PAF and phospholipase A_2, can cause or augment lung injury (19,20), which is characterized by cellular infiltration, increased permeability alveolar-capillary edema, hyaline membrane formation and surfactant dysfunction. However, the precise mechanisms responsible for the pathogenesis of ARDS are still vague. It is suggested that, PLase A_2 could be the major regulator which leads to the onset and evolution of ARDS.

In previous studies, we observed qualitative and quantitative disorders in BAL surfactant phospholipids during ARDS evolution, whereas phosphatidylcholine levels were correlated with the clinical outcome of the patients (16). The aim of the present study was, the determination of Ca^{2+}-dependent PLase A_2 and PAF-AcH activities in bronchoalveolar lavage (BAL) fluids of ARDS patients, the study of the balance between the activities for both enzymes, as well as the investigation of total activities distribution in bronchoalveolar lavage subfractions.

Materials and Methods

Material

BSA, EDTA, Tris-HCl and inorganic compounds were purchased from Sigma Chemical Co (St. Louis, USA). C_6-NBD-PC, C_6-NBD-FA, C_{12}-NBD-PC and C_{12}-NBD-FA were purchased from Avanti Polar Lipids (Pelham, AL, USA).

Patients and BAL procedure

Thirty one mechanically ventilated patients were used in this study. Twenty mechanically ventilated patients diagnosed with ARDS were studied. Eleven patients without cardiopulmonary disease were used as the control group. Bronchoalveolar lavage was performed by fiberoptic bronchoscopy, as described in a previous study. Patients were ventilated with a control mechanical ventilation mode. Six aliquots of 20 mL sterile normal saline at 37 °C were infused through the working channel of the bronchoscope. The first aspirated fluid, reflecting a bronchial sample, underwent microbiological screening, while the others were collected in ice-cold tubes. Bronchoalveolar lavage was filtered through sterile gauze so as mucus to be removed and then it was centrifuged at 500 x g for 15 min at 4 °C. The resulting pellet corresponded to BAL cells. The supernatant of 500 x g (BAL) was used for the determination of the enzymic activities.

Differential centrifugations of BAL/Isolation of surfactant subtypes

Lung surfactant was obtained in bronchoalveolar lavage (BAL) fluid. After BAL was subjected to ultra-centrifugations, surfactant were fractionated into different subtypes, the "heavy", "light" and "ultra-light" fractions. The "heavy" fraction comprise large surfactant aggregates (LSA) and consists mainly of lamellar bodies, tubular myelin and large multilamellar vesicles. The "light" as well as the "ultra-light" fractions which appear as small or very small unilamellar vesicles, contain the small (SSA) and very small surfactant aggregates (VSSA), respectively. LSA fractions generate the phospholipid monolayer on the alveolar-epithelium surface while SSA and VSSA are recycled by the alveolar type II cells or phagocytosed by the alveolar macrophages. Large surfactant aggregates are considered to be highly surface active while small and very small surfactant aggregates display poor surface activity (21).

Four representative BAL samples of ARDS patients and two control samples were subjected to ultra centrifugations for the isolation of surfactant subtypes. An aliquot ranging from 20 to 25 mL of the 500 g supernatant (BAL) was further centrifuged at 30,000 g at 4°C for 1 h (Beckman L5 ± 65B with NVT65 rotor). The pellet of 30,000 g (P30) which corresponds to large surfactant aggregates (LSA), was suspended in 3–5 mL of natural saline at 4 °C. The supernatant of 30,000 g was then submitted to ultracentrifugation at 100,000 g at 4 °C, for 1 h (Beckman L5 ± 65B with NVT65 rotor). The 100,000 g pellet (P100) which corresponds to small surfactant aggregates (SSA), was treated similarly to P30 and both were kept at –20 °C until the analysis of total proteins and the determination of phospholipases A_2 enzymic activities, as described below. The supernatant of 100,000 g (S100), representing the very small surfactant aggregates (VSSA) was also stored at –20 °C until further experimental use.

Protein measurement

Proteins was measured in BAL, in surfactant subfractions according to Lowry et al using bovine serum albumin as reference compound (22).

Phospholipase A_2 / PAF-AcH fluorimetric assay

Phospholipases A_2 enzymic activities were measured in BAL fluid and fractionated BAL with the application of the fluorimetric method developed by Kitsiouli et al (23). According to that, the fluorescent C_{12}-NBD-phosphatidylcholine and C_6-NBD-phosphatidylcholine were used as substrates for the determination of phospholipase A_2 and PAF-AcH activities, respectively.

Ten mM Tris-HCl buffer solution pH 7.4, 2 mM Ca^{2+} was used for the determination of phospholipase A_2 and 10 mM Tris-HCl buffer solution, 10 mM EDTA for the determination of PAF-AcH activity. The buffer volume, which was added to the cuvette initially, ranged between 890 and 980 μL. The addition of 10 μL of 0.5 mM of the C_{12}- or C_6-NBD-PC substrate (ethanol solution) and gentle agitation followed. In this step, the fluorescence was recorded and regarded as the initial substrate fluorescence.

At zero time, a volume of 10 to 100 μL of the source of the enzyme (or 5–100 μg of total protein) was added in the cuvette and the mixture was immediately agitated. The mixture was incubated at 28 °C for the reaction to occur. In 30 min of reaction time, we recorded the level of the fluorescence intensity of the solution (475 and 535 nm were the excitation and emission wavelengths, respectively). In different time intervals and every 15 min, approximately, the fluorescence intensity of the reaction mixture was measured. The total reaction time ranged between 1 ½ to 3 hours. Amidst fluorescence measurements, the reaction mixture had not been subjected to continuous excitation by the fluorimeter light beam. After the last measurement, internal standard was used with the addition of 2 μL of 0.1 mM C_{12}- or C_6-NBD-fatty acid ethanol solution three repeated times, for the following conversion of the fluorescence arbitrary units to nmol of the reaction product. A plot of the fluorescence intensity as a function of time (in minutes) was drawn and the best linear fit was made. The slope of the curve corresponded to the product formation. The lower detection limit of the method was estimated at 100 pmol of C_6- or C_{12}-NBD-fatty acid per hour. The enzymic activity was calculated with the use of the following equations:

$$EA_{(mL)} = \frac{6 \times S \times 10^4}{F \times V} \quad \text{or} \quad EA_{(p)} = \frac{6 \times S \times 10^7}{F \times V \times P}$$

where

$EA_{(mL)}$, (nmoles of NBD-fatty acid / mL /h):	Enzymic activity expressed in nmoles of liberated C_{12}- or C_6-NBD-fatty acid per mL of sample per hour
$EA_{(p)}$, (nmoles of NBD-fatty acid / mg protein /h):	Enzymic activity expressed in nmoles of liberated C_{12}- or C_6-NBD-fatty acid per mg of sample protein per hour
S, (Slope):	Slope of the curve of the fluorescence enhancement of the reaction mixture versus time (in minutes)
F, (NBD-fatty acid fluorescence):	Relative fluorescence of 1 nmole of the NBD-fatty acid in the presence of the reaction mixture components

V, (μL): Volume of the sample added

P, (μg/mL): Protein content of the sample expressed in μg of proteins per mL

Results

Phospholipase A_2 and PAF-acetylhydrolase levels in BAL

Both PLase A_2 and PAF-AcH enzymic activities were detected in high levels in BAL fluids of ARDS patients as compared to control group. The mean PLase A_2 activity measured in BAL fluid was 1.72 (± 1.37) and 0.16 (± 0.08) nmoles of C_{12}-NBD-FA / mL BAL / h for ARDS patients and control group, respectively (p=0.002, Figure 1).

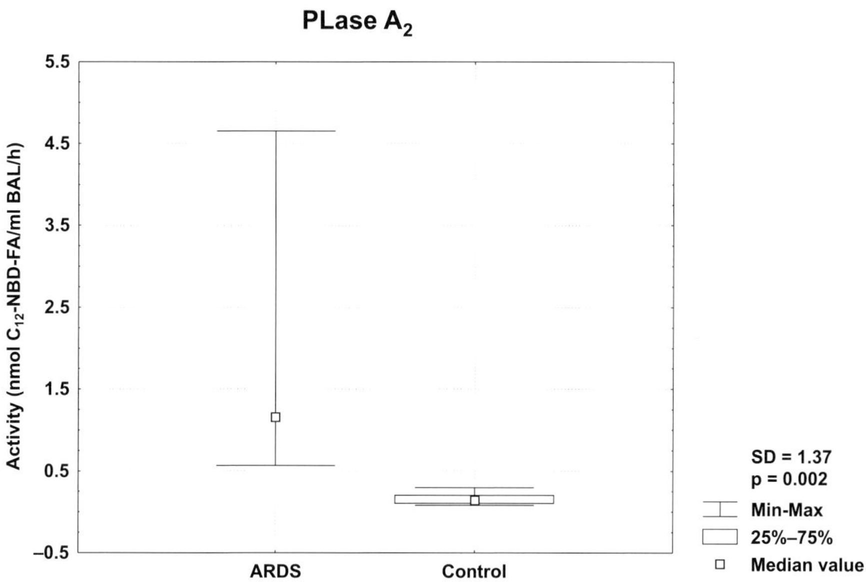

Figure 1. Phospholipase A_2 levels in bronchoalveolar lavage of patients with ARDS and control samples.

The mean PAF-AcH activity levels reached at 5.82 (± 4.47) in ARDS samples and 1.27 (± 0.80) in BAL fluids of the control group, all expressed in nmoles of C_6-NBD-FA / mL BAL / h (p=0.002, Figure 2).

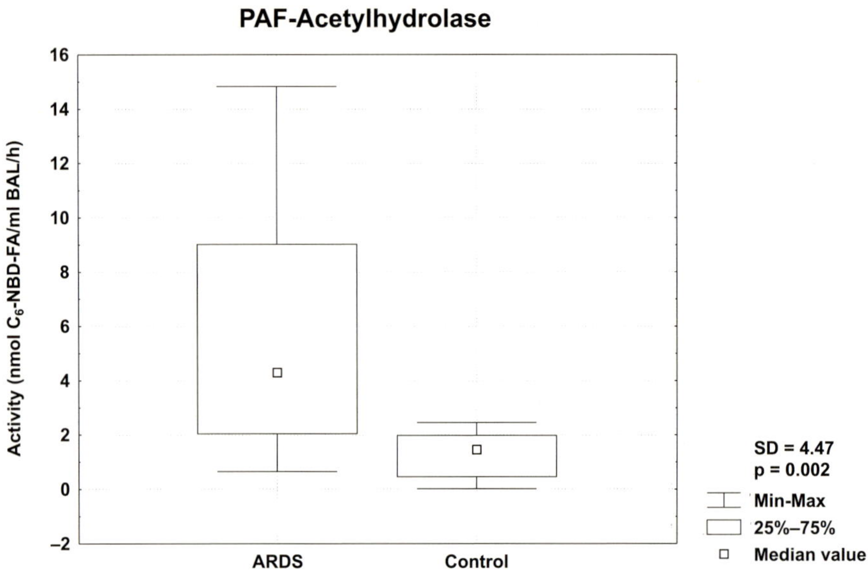

Figure 2. PAF-acetylhydrolase levels in bronchoalveolar lavage of patients with ARDS and control samples.

Phospholipase A_2 distribution in BAL subfractions

The distribution profile of the total PLase A_2 enzymic activity in BAL subfractions was the following: 37 (± 12) % of the total PLase A_2 activity was detected in the pellet of 30,000 g, 1 (± 1) % in the pellet of 100,000 g and 62 (± 11) % in the supernatant of 100,000 g, of BAL fluids from ARDS patients (Table 1, Figure 3). On the contrary, in two representative control BAL samples subjected to ultra centrifugations, it was indicated that the distribution of PLase A_2 activity differed from the previous one for ARDS patients. Despite the fact that, the detected PLase A_2 activities were very low, compared to ARDS samples, the higher percentage (72 %) was measured in the pellet of 30,000 g while the 2.4 % and 26 % of the rest enzymic activity was detected in the pellet of 100,000 g and supernatant of 100,000 g, respectively.

Table 1. PLase A_2 and PAF-AcH total activities distribution in surfactant subfractions of ARDS and control patients.

BAL subfractions	***Total enzymic activities in ARDS***	
	PLase A_2 nmoles of C_{12}-NBD-FA/h	**PAF-AcH nmoles of C_6-NBD-FA/h**
P30 (Large surfactant aggregates)	5.3 ± 3.4	19.5 ± 7.6
P100 (Small surfactant aggregates)	0.2 ± 0.3	8.2 ± 4.6
S100 (Very small surfactant aggregates)	9.1 ± 6.8	33.3 ± 15.0

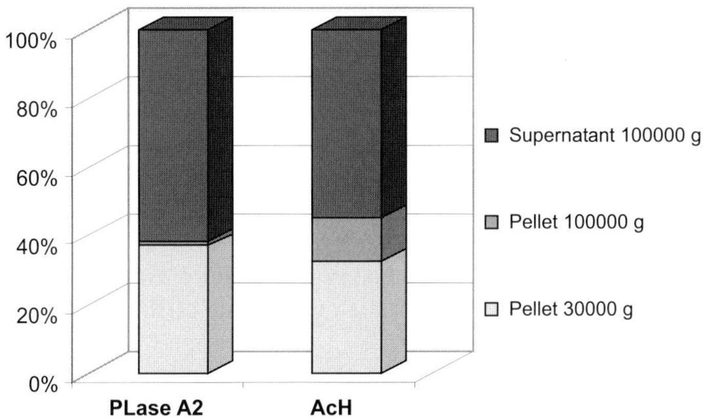

Figure 3. Total enzymic activities distribution in BAL subfractions of ARDS patients.

PAF-acetylhydrolase distribution in BAL subfractions

Similarly with PLase A_2, the higher percentage of PAF-AcH total activity of BAL fluids from ARDS patients was distributed in the supernatant of 100,000 g. Thus, 33 (± 11), 12 (± 3) and 55 (± 12) % of the total activity was found in the P30, P100 and S100 fractions of BAL from ARDS patients, respectively (Table 1, Figure 3). However, no significant differences were observed in the distribution of the total PAF-AcH activity between ARDS samples and the control samples.

Discussion

In the present study, Ca^{2+}-dependent phospholipases A_2 and PAF-acetylhydrolase activities were measured in bronchoalveolar lavage fluid and its subfractions from ARDS patients and control subjects. The determination was assessed by a fluorimetric method developed by Kitsiouli et al, in which NBD-phosphatidylcholine analogues were used as substrates. Increased levels of Ca^{2+}-dependent phospholipase A_2 and PAF-acetylhydrolase activities were detected in high levels of BAL fluid of patients with ARDS as compared to control group. Considering the total activities, in ARDS patients the highest percentage of both Ca^{2+}-dependent PLase A_2 and PAF-AcH were found in the supernatant of 100,000 g (S100). However, in the control group, PLase A_2 total activity was distributed in the 30,000 g pellet (P30), whereas PAF-AcH was located in the S100 fraction.

BAL fluid represents alveolar fluid in dilution (24). In healthy subjects it contains low levels of protein, while different formations of lung surfactant are recovered during the lavage. These include large surfactant aggregates (LSA), which can exhibit an efficient depression in the surface tension within the alveolar space, as well as small (SSA) and very small vesicles (VSSA), which are insufficient for this role. Alveolar macrophages are the dominant cellular components. During the course of ARDS, proteinaceous edema fluid floods into the alveolar space, different inflammatory mediators appear and a recruitment of cells, most often neutrophils, takes place. The ratio of small to large aggregates is increased (25).

In the present study, in BAL fluid of ARDS patients, a Ca^{2+}-dependent PLase A_2 was identified in significantly higher levels when compared to control group. Our findings agree with other studies, in which the critical role of this enzyme is supported.

Kim et al found that PLase A_2 activities in BAL fluid of patients with ARDS were correlated with the severity of lung injury. In this study, the substrates of phosphatidylcholine and phosphatidylethanolamine esterified with arachidonic acid at the *sn*-2 position were used. On the contrary, others investigators had failed to detect PLase A_2 activity in BAL (26,27). Kim et al. attributed these results to the lower PLase A_2 activity on substrates with fatty acyl chain at the *sn*-2 position shorter than arachidonic acid. Nevertheless, our results clearly display the existence of Ca^{2+}-dependent PLase A_2 activity in BAL fluid of ARDS patients, for the first time with the substrate of C_{12}-NBD-PC. This fluorescent phospholipid seems to be a substrate analogue to dipalmitoyl-PC, since it disposes similar polarity as it was shown by TLC analysis of both phospholipids, in which C_{12}-NBD-PC and C_{12}-NBD-FA migrate at the same R_f with dipalmitoyl-PC and palmitic acid, respectively.

PLase A_2 activity can be detrimental in the lungs because it can hydrolyze lung surfactant phospholipids (28,29). Surfactant alterations as well as deficient surfactant function lead to alveolar collapse, a loss of liquid balance in the lung and of local defense mechanism and finally acute respiratory distress syndrome (30).

PLase A_2 enzyme could be produced locally and secreted into the alveolar space from the inflammatory cells, or it could derive from circulation, due to increased alveolar-capillary permeability. The alveolar macrophages have been reported as the major source of this enzyme in the lungs (31). However, various cell types, such as platelets, mast cells, fibroblasts, macrophages and neutrophils, synthesize and secrete phospholipase A_2 following stimulation (32).

PAF-AcH activity levels were higher in BAL fluid of ARDS patients when compared to control subjects. In this syndrome, increased levels of PAF had been detected as well in ARDS. In the case of high-pressure pulmonary edema an inverse correlation of PAF/PAF-AcH has only been identified. The parallel increase of PAF-AcH and PAF in ARDS suggests that PAF-AcH mainly derives from serum, due to increased alveolar-capillary permeability. However, alveolar macrophages could produce locally and secrete this enzyme in the alveolar space. Clinical studies have focused on the administration of recombinant PAF-AcH to patients at risk for developing the acute respiratory distress syndrome (ARDS), in order to control or attenuate inflammation (33).

The higher percentage of the total amount of PLase A_2 as well as PAF-AcH activity were detected in the supernatant of 100,000 g. In this fraction of BAL, small vesicles which do not contribute in lowering surface tension at the water/air interface of the alveolar epithelium are recovered. It is known that, the ratio of small to large surfactant aggregates is significantly increased in patients with ARDS compared to non-ARDS patients. Conversion of surfactant large aggregates into small aggregates in BAL of ARDS patients results in reduction of SP-B levels in large aggregates and this reduction is correlated with the loss of surface activity (34). Thus, the presence of PLase A_2 in this fraction of BAL could play a role on the deactivation and disorganization of the surface-active forms of surfactant, can lead to surfactant deficiency and could contribute to the development of respiratory failure.

The activities of PLase A_2 and PAF-AcH were measured fluorimetrically, with C_{12}- and C_6-NBD-phosphatidylcholine as substrates, respectively. The capability of PAF-AcH to cleave C_6-NBD-PC had been also found during the investigation of the enzymic activities that mediate PC hydrolysis during LDL oxidation (35). With the present fluorimetric method we can get information for a wide spectrum of phospholipase A_2 activities, whether it concerns hydrolysis of long-fatty acid esterified phopholipids, or PAF or oxidized phospholipids. The method is applicable either in lipid-rich or on lipid-poor physicochemical environments.

In conclusion, PLase A_2 and PAF-AcH could play important role in the development or down-regulation of inflammation in ARDS, respectively. With the proposed fluorimetric method, both PLase A_2 and PAF-AcH activities can be measured in varying water/lipid environments. The sensitivity of the method is very high, comparable to that of radiometric methods (100 pmoles of product per hour). In addition, the sample volume required is very low (under 100 μL). The method was found sufficient and reproducible for measuring both the enzymic activities in BAL fluid or surfactant subfractions of ARDS patients.

References

1. Gijon, M.A. and Leslie, C.C., Phospholipases A_2. *Semin Cell Dev Biol, 1997; 8: 297–303.*
2. Balsinde, J., Balboa, M.A., Inset, P.A. and Dennis, E.A. Regulation and inhibition of phospholipase A_2. *Annu Rev Pharmacol Toxicol, 1999; 39: 175–189.*
3. Capper EA, Marshall LA. Mammalian phospholipases A_2: mediators of inflammation, proliferation and apoptosis. *Progress Lipid Res, 2001; 40: 167–197.*
4. Six DA, Dennis EA. The expanding superfamily of phospholipase A_2 enzymes: classification and characterization. *Biochim Biophys Acta, 2000; 1488: 1–19.*
5. Tjoelker, L.W., Wilder, C., Eberhardt, C., Stafforini, D.M., Dietsch, G., Schimpf, B., Hooper, S., Le Trong, H., Cousens, L.S., Zimmerman, G.A. et al., Anti-inflammatory properties of a platelet-activating factor acetylhydrolase. *Nature, 1995; 374: 549–553.*
6. Derewenda ZS, Ho YS. PAF-acetylhydrolases. *Biochim Biophys Acta 1999; 1441: 229–236.*
7. Hite RD, Seeds MC, Jacinto RB, Balasubramanian R, Waite M, Bass D. Hydrolysis of surfactant-associated phosphatidylcholine by mammalian secretory phospholipase A_2. *Am J Physiol 1998; 275: L740–L747.*
8. Holm BA, Keicher L, Liu MY, Sokolowski J, Enhorning G. Inhibition of pulmonary surfactant function by phospholipases. *J Appl Physiol 1991; 71: 317–321.*
9. Matsumoto K, Taki F, Kondoh Y, Taniguchi H, Takagi K. Platelet activating factor in bronchoalveolar lavage fluid of patients with adult respiratory distress syndrome. *Clin Exp Pharmacol Physiol 1992; 19: 509–515.*
10. Kim DK, Fukuda T, Thompson BT, Cockrill B, Hales C, Bonventre JV. Bronchoalveolar lavage fluid phospholipase A_2 activities are increased in human adult respiratory distress syndrome. *Am J Physiol 1995; 269: L109–L118.*
11. Takahide Nagase, Naonori Uozumi, Satoshi Ishii, Kazuhiko Kume, Takashi Izumi, Yasuyoshi Ouchi and Takao Shimizu. Acute lung injury by sepsis and acid aspiration: a key role for cytosolic phospholipase A_2. *Nature Immunol 2000; 1: 42–46.*
12. Romaschin AD, DeMajo WC, Winton T, D'Costa M, Chang G, Rubin B, GamLiel Z, Walker PM, Systemic phospholipase A_2 and cachectin levels in adult respiratory distress syndrome and multiple-organ failure. *Clin Biochem 1992; 25: 55–60.*
13. Nyman KM, Uhl W, Forsstrom J, Buchler M, Beger HG, Nevalainen TJ. Serum phospholipase A_2 in patients with multiple organ failure. *J Surg Res 1996, 60: 7–14.*
14. Sorensen J, Kald B, Tagesson C, Lindahl M. Platelet-activating factor and phospholipase A_2 in patients with septic shock and trauma. *Int Care Med 1994; 20: 553–561.*
15. Triggiani M, De Marino V, Sofia M, Faraone S, Ambrosio G, Carratu L, Marone G. Characterization of platelet-activating factor acetylhydrolase in human bronchoalveolar lavage. *Am J Resp Crit Care Med 1997; 156: 94–100.*
16. Nakos, G., E.I. Kitsiouli, I. Tsangaris, M.E. Lekka. Bronchoalveolar lavage fluid characteristics of early intermediate and late phases of ARDS. Alterations in leukocytes, proteins, PAF and surfactant components. *Intensive Care Med., 1998; 24(4): 296–303.*
17. Nakos G, Kitsiouli E., Lekka ME. Bronchoalveolar lavage alterations in pulmonary embolism. *Am J Resp Crit Care Med 1998; 155: 945–950.*
18. Nakos G, Pneumatikos J, Tsangaris H, Tellis K, Lekka ME. Protein and phospholipids in BAL from patients with hydrostatic pulmonary edema. *Am J Resp Crit Care Med 1997; 155: 945–951.*
19. Touqui, L. and Arbibe, L., A role for phospholipase A_2 in ARDS pathogenesis. *Mol. Med. Today, 1999; 5: 244–249.*
20. Anderson B, Moore EE, Banerjee A. Phospholipase A_2 regulates critical inflammatory mediators of multiple organ failure. *J Surg Res 1994; 56: 199–205.*
21. Magoon MW, Wright A, Baritussio M, Williams J, Goerke BJ, Benson RL, Hamilton Clements JA. Sufractionation of lung surfactant. Implications for metabolism and surface activity. *Biochim Biophys Acta 1983, 750: 18–31.*

22. Lowry OH, Rosebrough NJ, Farr AL, Randall RJ. Protein measurement with the Folin phenol reagent. *J Biol Chem 1951; 193: 265–275.*
23. Kitsiouli EI, Nakos G, Lekka ME. Differential determination of phospholipase A_2 and PAF-acetylhydrolase in biological fluids using fluorescent substrates. *J Lipid Res 1999; 40(12): 2346–2356.*
24. Reynolds HY. Bronchoalveolar lavage. *Am Rev Respir Dis 1987; 135: 250–263.*
25. Veldhuizen RAW, McCaig LA, Akino T, Lewis JF. Pulmonary surfactant subfractions in patients with the acute respiratory distress syndrome. *Am J Respir Crit Care Med 1995; 152: 1867–1871.*
26. Zhou W, McColum MO, Levine BA, Olson MS. Role of platelet-activating factor in pancreatitis-associated acute lung injury in the rat. *Am J Pathol 1992; 140: 971–979.*
27. Casals C, Herrera L, Miguel E, Garcia-Barreno P, Municio A. Comparison between intra- and extracellular surfactant in respiratory distress induced by oleic acid. *Biochim Biophys Acta 1989; 1003: 201–203.*
28. Duncan JE, Hatch GM, Belik J. Susceptibility of exogenous surfactant to phospholipase A_2 degradation. *Can J Physiol Pharmacol 1996; 74: 957–963.*
29. Arbibe L, Koumanov K, Vial D, Rougeot C, Faure G, Havet N, Longacre S, Vargaftig BB, Berezliat G, Voelker DR, Wolf C, Touqui L. Generation of lyso-phospholipids from surfactant in acute lung injury is mediated by type-II phospholipase A_2 and inhibited by a direct surfactant protein A-phospholipase A_2 protein interaction. *J Clin Invest 1998; 102: 1152–1160.*
30. Hamm H, Kroegel C, Hohlfeld J. Surfactant: a review of its functions and relevance in adult respiratory disorders. *Respir Med 1996; 90: 251–270.*
31. Arbibe L, Vial D, RosinskiChupin I, Havet N, Huerre M, Vargaftig BB, Touqui L. Endotoxin induces expression of type II phospholipase A_2 in macrophages during acute lung injury in guinea pigs: involvement of TNF-alpha in lipopolydacharide-induced type II phospholipase A_2 synthesis. *J Immunol 1997; 159: 391–400.*
32. Nevalainen TJ, Haapamaki MM, Gronroos JM. Roles of phospholipases A_2 in inflammatory diseases and trauma. *Biochim Biophys Acta 2000; 1488: 83–90.*
33. Metzler M, Balk R, Schuster D, Slotman G, Michael J, Zimmerman J, Coyne E, Pribble. An evaluation of recombinant human platelet-activating factor acetylhydrolase (rPAF-AH) in patients at risk for developing acute respiratory distress syndrome (ARDS). *Crit Care Med 1999; 27 (Suppl. 1): 85A.*

Günther A, Schmidt R, Feustel A, Meier U, Pucker C, Ermert M, Seeger W. Surfactant subtype conversion is related to loss of surfactant apoprotein B and surface activity in large surfactant aggregates. *Am J Respir Crit Care Med 1999; 159: 244–251*

UP Steinbrecher,Pritchard PH. Hydrolysis of phosphatidylcholine during LDL oxidation is mediated by platelet-activating factor acetylhydrolase. J Lipid Res 1989: 30: 305–315.

BLOOD GASES – ELECTROLYTES – TRACE ELEMENTS

National Winner

Magnesium In The ICU

A. Abraham, A. Bachwani

Parsee General Hospital, Mumbai, INDIA.

Abtract

Introduction

Magnesium has been used in the past as a purgative & uterine relaxant. Magnesium regulates many life processes & is the key factor in the production of ATP, the source of life energy. It is also a natural Calcium channel blocker and neutralizes the effect of catecholamines. We obtained excellent results on cardiac arrhythmias and drug induced supraventricular tachycardia. The aim of this study is to evaluate the effects of Magnesium in different critical settings.

Methods

Five gms of Magnesium was administered in D5W over 6–8 hours. The heart rate was monitored at 15, 30, 45, 60, 75 & 90 min & then at 6 & 12-hour interval. The same dose was given for five consecutive days keeping a vigil on other parameters like urine output, creatinine and patient outcome.

Results

Case Control study: 115 cases treated with Magnesium (50-drug induced SVT, 20-SVT, 5-ARDS, 16-CCF, 7-CPR, 7-Diabetic Ketoacidosis, 1-Carpopedal Spasm, 1-Hypokalemia induced by the Chronic Alcoholism.

The following are the average heart rates observed after administering magnesium:

0 min	15 min	30 min	45 min	60 min	75 min	90 min	6 hours	12 hours
164	138	129	108	101	100	96	92	94

Patho	No of pat.	Heart Rate	Urine output	Creatinine	Died	Surv
Drug induced	51	164–108/mnt	Improved	Not studied	Not studied	Not studied
SVT	20	180–84/mnt (45mnt)	Improved	Normal	0	20
ARDS	5	130–84/mnt	Improved	Reduced	3	2
CCF	16	144–102/mnt	Improved	7–1	8	8
CPR	8	Vent. Tach. -Norm. rhythm	Improved	Not studied	2	6
DKA	78	150–96/mnt	Improved	Reduced (N)	2	5

Carpopedal Spasm was relieved after magnesium was given in one case & a chronic alcohol abuse induced hypokalemia was rectified too. Base deficit came to normal in 4–5 hours.

Conclusions

1. Tachycardia induced by inotropes or cardiac pathology decreases to an acceptable rate when magnesium is given within an average of 45 minutes.
2. Patients were conferred cyto protection from Tachyarrhythmias. Incidences of drug-induced arrhythmias when magnesium was given concomitantly with inotropes or bronchodilators like aminophyline are nil.
3. Magnesium improves energy production (ATP) & stimulates metabolism. This is advantageous as patients requiring ionotropes are always in shock.
4. The effect of magnesium therapy on Base Deficit (Lactic Acidosis) needs to be studied, because of the encouraging normal base values observed within 5–6 hours after magnesium was given.

CARDIOLOGY – HAEMODYNAMICS – STROKE

Finalist

Single-Point Troponin T Measurement On The Day Of Coronary Care Unit Discharge After Myocardial Infarction Strongly Correlates With Ejection Fraction And Infarct Size By Nuclear Imaging And With CK-MB Release

G. Bonetti, F. Pagani, R. Giubbini, C. Cuccia, M. Panteghini

Azienda Ospedaliera 'Spedali Civili', Brescia, ITALY

Abstract

Introduction

The extent of injury to the myocardium after infarction – one of the most influential factors in the prognosis – has previously been assessed by CK-MB release curves using serial serum sampling(1). Aim of the present study was to investigate the ability of a single-point measurement of circulating cardiac troponin T (cTnT) concentrations, performed on day of discharge from coronary care unit (CCU), to estimate the infarct size and assess left ventricular (LV) function in patients with acute myocardial infarction (AMI).

Methods

We studied 51 patients with AMI presenting 4.0 hours (range: 0.5–41 hours) after the onset of chest pain. LV function was evaluated by gated single-photon emission computed tomography (SPECT) imaging and infarct size was estimated by CK-MB peak concentrations and SPECT myocardial perfusion using technetium 99m-sestamibi. Measurements of cTnT, on a single fresh EDTA sample, and SPECT were performed in the morning on the day of CCU discharge (median time after admission: 72 hours, range: 40–160). Serum samples for CK-MB peak estimation were taken every 6 hours throughout the first 48 hours after admission. cTnT and CK-MB mass concentrations were measured on the Elecsys system (Roche Diagnostics).

Results

The perfusion defect sizes at SPECT, expressed as % of left ventricle, ranged from 0% to 63% (median, 19%) and the LV ejection fractions (LVEF) ranged from 22% to 58% (median, 42%). A significant positive correlation was found between plasma cTnT concentrations (median 2.22 mg/L, range 0.18–7.55) and both the peak CK-MB concentration ($r=0.76$, $p<0.001$) and the perfusion defect size at SPECT ($r=0.57$, $p<0.001$). As expected, a close correlation between CK-MB peaks and scintigraphic defect sizes ($r=0.66$, $p<0.001$) was also found. cTnT concentrations were inversely related to LVEF ($r=-0.50$, $p<0.001$) and positively correlated with LV end-systolic and end-diastolic volumes ($r=0.57$, $p<0.001$, and $r=0.50$, $p<0.001$, respectively). A cTnT concentration of >2.27 mg/L predicted a LVEF of <40% with a sensitivity of 81.8% [95% confidence interval (CI): 59.7–94.7] and specificity of 82.1% (CI: 63.1–93.9). Analysis by ROC curve produced an area under curve of 0.821 (CI: 0.687–0.915).

Conclusions

A single measurement of plasma cTnT concentrations on the day of CCU discharge after AMI, regardless of the kinetic of marker appearance in blood, can be used as a convenient and cost-effective, non-invasive estimate of infarct size and for the assessment of LV function in routine clinical setting, revealing a similar reliability as peak CK-MB measurement (requiring however repetitive sampling) or nuclear imaging (too expensive to be routinely used). Since the major concern about totally replacing CK-MB with cardiac troponins in hospital institutions is the lack of evidence on the ability of troponins to estimate the AMI size (2), our findings support the definitive implementation of cTnT testing and the replacement of CK-MB in the laboratory cardiac panel.

References

1. Christenson RH, Vollmer RT, Ohman EM et al. Relation of temporal creatine kinase-MB release and outcome after thrombolytic therapy for acute myocardial infarction. Am J Cardiol 2000;85: 543–7.
2. Wu AHB, Apple FS, Gibler WB et al. National Academy of Clinical Biochemistry Standards of Laboratory Practice: Recommendations for the use of cardiac markers in coronary artery diseases. Clin Chem 1999;45: 1104–21.

Introduction

The evaluation of infarct size after acute myocardial infarction (AMI) is important for predicting the subsequent clinical course and to validate the effectiveness and clinical relevance of therapeutic interventions (1–3). Quantitative histologic estimates of infarct size are regarded as the gold standard but obviously this technique has little clinical relevance. It is rather desirable to find a simple and reliable method with which to quantify infarct size (4,5). In case of need, a variety of techniques, such as electrocardiography, echocardiography, left ventriculography, radionuclide methods, and the release of cardiac biomarkers, have been proposed (6).

In clinical practice, the extent of injury to the myocardium after AMI is generally assessed by creatine kinase isoenzyme MB (CK-MB) release curves using serial serum sampling (7,8). Although quantitative calculations using area under the CK-MB vs time curve are seldom made, many physicians use peak CK-MB to get a qualitative estimate as to the AMI size (9,10). The well-known limitations of CK-MB measurement, such as short duration of elevation following AMI, requiring repetitive, frequent sampling for evaluation of peak concentrations, and sensitivity to reperfusion status, as well as lack of specificity for cardiac damage, have however stimulated the search for a more suitable biomarker for sizing AMI (11).

Cardiac troponin T (cTnT) is a cardiac-specific protein that is compartmented in the contractile apparatus of the myocardial cell. Its release process into the blood after myocardial injury is slow (cTnT is present in plasma for more than 120 hours after AMI) and slightly affected by reperfusion of the infarct zone (12). For these characteristics, plasma cTnT has been used for the estimation of infarct size in animals (13–16). In humans, only two clinical studies have examined the correlation of plasma cTnT release to infarct size, both using serial measurements to calculate cTnT peak concentrations and area under cTnT curves (17–18). However, in clinical practice serial analyses are not feasible.

In a well-conducted experimental study, Remppis et al (15). first demonstrated the usefulness of cTnT determined at a fixed time point, i.e. 96 hours, after the onset of AMI for a noninvasive estimation of infarct size in dogs. In the present study, we investigated the ability of a *single-point* measurement of circulating cTnT concentrations, performed on the day of discharge from coronary care unit (CCU), to estimate the infarct size and assess left ventricular (LV) function in AMI patients, in comparison with parameters obtained from gated single-photon emission computed tomography (SPECT) imaging. For the biochemical assessment of infarct size, CK-MB release was also studied.

Methods

Patients

Sixty five patients with AMI (58 men and seven women; median age, 53 years, range 24–78) who were admitted to our CCU between May 2000 and June 2001 were prospectively enrolled for this study. These were not consecutive admissions, but no conscious bias was applied in their selection. We included patients who satisfied all the following criteria: (1) typical serial changes of serum CK-MB mass concentrations and electrocardiographic evidence of AMI, (2) hospitalization within 20 hours after the onset of symptoms, (3) no evidence of prior AMI, and (4) informed consent to allow an extra blood sample for cTnT to be drawn at CCU discharge and underwent SPECT imaging. The diagnosis of AMI was made in each patient by a cardiologist without access to cTnT or scintigraphic results. The approximate anatomic region of AMI was determined by electrocardiogram (ECG).

Forty seven patients sustained an anterior and 18 an inferior wall AMI. On admission (median time from symptom onset: 4.5 hours, range 0.5–19), all but two patients, showing left bundle branch block, showed ST-segment elevation or depression of 0.1 mV or more in at least two contiguous leads at ECG. Subsequently, new persistent Q waves developed in 39 (60%) patients. 55 (84.6%) patients underwent revascularization: 15 received intravenous thrombolytic therapy, 28 primary percutaneous transluminal coronary angioplasty, and 12 both. The remaining 10 patients were treated with conventional therapy. Except for a patient who suddenly died of a subarachnoid hemorrhage two weeks after admission, all patients had an uncomplicated AMI course (no reinfarction) throughout the study period.

Protocol

Serial venous blood (serum) samples for CK-MB peak estimation were taken every 6 hours throughout the first 48 hours after CCU admission. In addition, for cTnT measurement, a single EDTA, tripotassium salt, blood sample was collected on the morning of day of CCU discharge (median time after admission: 72 hours, range: 40–160). Blood samples were centrifuged immediately and biochemical assays were performed without delay.

At the same time of blood collection for cTnT assay, LV function and infarct size were evaluated by gated SPECT imaging. A further SPECT estimation of LV function was performed in 58 of the enrolled patients about three months after hospital discharge. Of the originally enrolled population, one patient died and 6 patients refused the repetition of SPECT procedure.

Laboratory assays

CK-MB mass concentrations were measured on an Elecsys® system (Roche Diagnostics). A previously calculated upper reference limit of 6 mg/L was used. Measurements of cTnT were carried out with the Elecsys analyzer using the third-generation assay (19). The detection limit of the assay is 0.01 µg/L and the decision limit used in our hospital for AMI diagnosis is 0.03 µg/L, i.e. the cTnT concentration that meets the imprecision goal of 10% total coefficient of variation (20,21).

We used CK-MB peak values as biochemical estimates of infarct size. A value was defined as a peak if it was the highest in the concentration time course and if we observed at least one lower value before and after a maximal level.

Scintigraphy

Scintigraphic estimation of infarct size using gated SPECT with technetium-99m sestamibi was performed in resting patients on the day of CCU discharge (22). Quantitative defect size as measurement of infarct size was expressed as percentage of total LV mass. Gated SPECT imaging also provided information on LV function. In particular, the LV ejection fraction (LVEF) was calculated by dividing the difference between LV end-diastolic volume (LVEDV) and LV end-systolic volume (LVESV) by LVEDV. A second SPECT study of LVEF was also performed approximately three months after hospital discharge of patients. Procedures and data analysis were performed by independent investigators with no knowledge of patient histories or the results of tests for biochemical markers.

Statistics

Median and range were calculated to describe continuous variables. Correlations were calculated using standard linear regression analysis. A probability (*P*) value of less than 0.05 was considered to be significant. Receiver operating characteristic (ROC) curves were constructed to examine the relation between cTnT concentration and LVEF. In this technique, the patients were categorized into two datasets, those with a LVEF of $< 40\%$ and those with a LVEF of $\geq 40\%$, producing a binary classification. The 40% LVEF cutoff was based on previous clinical trials as having prognostic significance (23,24). The ability of cTnT to assign AMI patients accurately into the two groups was determined by calculating the area under the curve (AUC). According to Swets' scheme for interpreting AUC (25), values from 0.5 to 0.7 indicate low diagnostic accuracy, values from 0.7 to 0.9 suggest limited clinical utility, and values greater than 0.9 mean high global diagnostic accuracy. The sensitivity, the specificity, and the likelihood ratio at the best decision value were also calculated. The 95% confidence intervals (CI) for the population proportions were calculated from the sample proportions by using the appropriate upper-tail probability. All statistical analyses were performed using MedCalcâ for Windows (MedCalc Software).

Results

In the patients studied, the perfusion defect sizes at SPECT, expressed as percentage of left ventricle, ranged from 0% to 63% (median, 21%) and LVEF in the acute phase ranged from 17% to 58% (median, 40%). CK-MB peak values ranged from 17 mg/L to 1323 mg/L, with a median value of 275 mg/L. A significant positive correlation was found between plasma cTnT concentrations (median 2.27 mg/L, range 0.04–7.55) and both the peak CK-MB concentration ($r=0.76$, $P<0.001$) (Figure 1) and the perfusion defect size at SPECT ($r=0.62$, $P<0.001$) (Figure 2). A close correlation between CK-MB peaks and scintigraphic defect sizes (r=0.66, $P<0.001$) was also found.

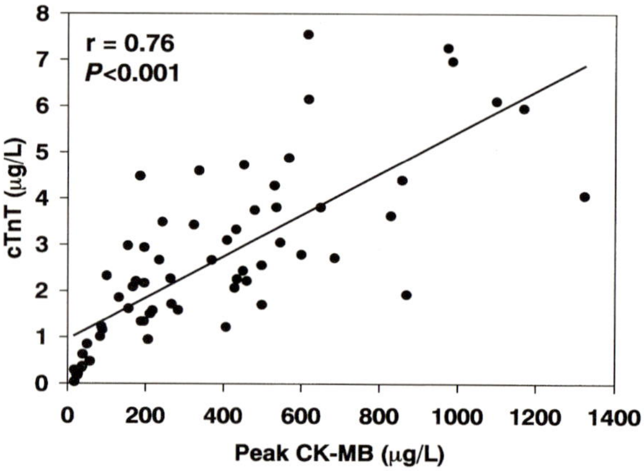

Figure 1. Correlation between cardiac troponin T (cTnT) concentrations at coronary care unit discharge and CK-MB concentrations at peak in the studied patients with acute myocardial infarction.

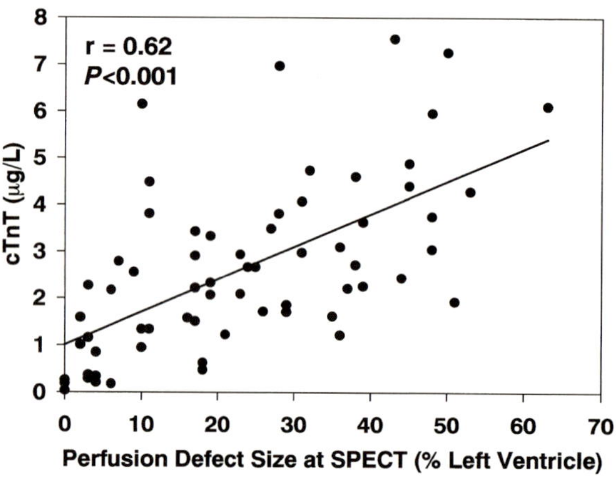

Figure 2. Correlation between cardiac troponin T (cTnT) concentrations and the scintigraphic estimate of infarct size, both measured at coronary care unit discharge, in the studied patients with acute myocardial infarction.

When the relation between cTnT and parameters of LV function at SPECT performed at time of CCU discharge was assessed, cTnT concentrations were inversely related to LVEF (r=–0.56, $P<0.001$) (Figure 3) and positively correlated with LVESV and LVEDV (r=0.58, $P<0.001$, and r=0.55, $P<0.001$, respectively). A cTnT concentration of >2.27 mg/L predicted a LVEF of <40% in the acute phase of AMI with a sensitivity of 82.8% (CI: 64.2–94.1), a specificity of 80.0% (CI: 63.1–91.5), and a likelihood ratio for a positive test of 4.1. Analysis by ROC curve produced an AUC (± SE) of 0.82 (CI: 0.71–0.91) ± 0.054, indicating the fairly good accuracy of cTnT in identifying patients with decreased LV function in the acute phase of AMI (Figure 4).

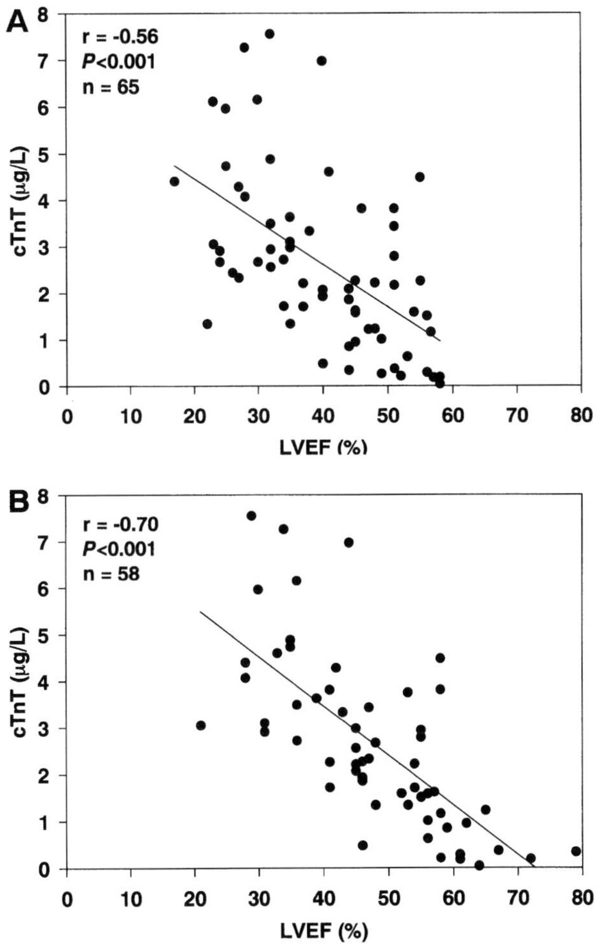

Figure 3. Correlation between cardiac troponin T (cTnT) concentrations at coronary care unit (CCU) discharge and the left ventricular ejection fraction (LVEF) assessed at CCU discharge (A) and three months after hospitalization (B) in the studied patients with acute myocardial infarction.

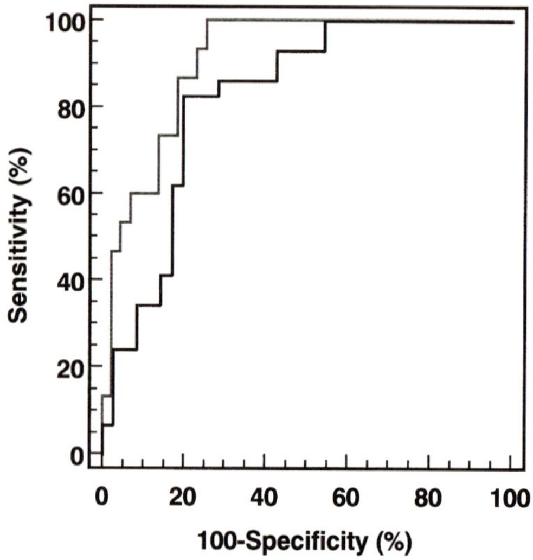

Figure 4. Receiver operating characteristic (ROC) curve analysis for cardiac troponin T measured at coronary care unit discharge as diagnostic test of left ventricular ejection fraction <40% in the acute phase of myocardial infarction (black line) and three months later (grey line) with the patient population studied.

Considering the relation between cTnT measured at CCU discharge and SPECT parameters obtained three months after AMI, the overall accuracy of cTnT in predicting LV function significantly increased. cTnT was still significantly related to LVEF (r=–0.70, *P*<0.001) (Figure 3) and the calculation of AUC gave a value of 0.91 (CI: 0.80–0.97) ± 0.053, indicating an excellent diagnostic accuracy of cTnT (Figure 4). In particular, a cTnT concentration of >2.98 mg/L predicted a LVEF of <40% at three months after AMI with a sensitivity of 86.7% (95% CI: 59.5–98.0), a specificity of 81.4% (95% CI: 66.6–91.6), and a likelihood ratio for a positive test of 4.7.

The results of re-analysis to examine the effect of revascularization by excluding the 10 patients who did not receive reperfusion therapy were no different from analysis of all patients.

Discussion

Estimation of the extent of myocardial injury from the release of CK-MB into plasma is a normal clinical practice (11). However, cardiac troponins have recently been proposed as new biochemical standard for diagnosis of AMI and, consequently, hospitals should consider the replacement of CK-MB measurement with this new marker at their institutions (20). One of the major concern about totally replacing CK-MB with cardiac troponins is just the lack of robust evidence on the ability of troponins to estimate the AMI size in clinical practice (26). Few studies have so far evaluated troponins as markers for assessment of infarct size in comparison with traditional serological markers and other techniques (17,18,27). Consequently, we decided to evaluate the ability of cTnT measurement to predict infarct size and LV function in patients with AMI admitted to CCU of our general hospital to support the definitive implementation of cTnT testing and the replacement of CK-MB assay in our laboratory cardiac panel. In particular, we evaluated the possibility to use a more advantageous single cTnT measurement, performed approximately at the time corresponding to the plateau phase of the release in blood, instead of previously used marker kinetics and peaks. Furthermore, the cTnT performance was consciously tested on a heterogeneous AMI population, irrespective of reperfusion status.

In our study, cTnT closely correlated with SPECT estimates of infarct size and peak serum concentrations of CK-MB. Our results corroborate those of earlier clinical studies, in which cTnT release, and not a single-point measurement, was however used to assess infarct size (17,18). Furthermore, our findings in living patients are consistent with those experimentally obtained in dogs by Remppis et al (15), who found a good correlation ($r=0.69$, $P=0.003$, $n=16$) between the cTnT levels 96 hours after the onset of ischemia and the pathoanatomical infarct size as quantified by the 2,3,5-triphenyltetrazolium chloride method. In clinical practice, the estimates of AMI size by cTnT determination on a single plasma sample at CCU discharge would facilitate the choice of appropriate degree of care, resulting in more efficient and economic use of the health care facilities. In fact, this approach appears to be more useful than analyzing cumulative cTnT release as previously proposed, due to the requirement of repetitive sampling and a possible incomplete recovery of cTnT (28).

LVEF is a very powerful prognostic indicator after AMI (23). A strong inverse relation exists between LV function and patient outcome, with a "break-point" at a LVEF of 40% and rapidly increasing mortality rates below that value (24). Rao et al (29) first showed a good correlation between cTnT concentration measured 12–48 hours after admission and LVEF ($r=-0.72$, $P<0.001$, $n=50$). In the study, a cTnT concentration of >2.8 µg/L predicted a LVEF of <40% with a sensitivity of 100% and specificity of 93% (AUC=0.98) (29). More recently, Kanna et al (30) confirmed that serum cTnT concentrations on day 3 or 4 after AMI had a significant negative correlation with LVEF assessed one month later ($r=-0.48$, $P<0.001$, $n=86$). No studies to date have however used gated SPECT imaging to assess LV function in comparison with cTnT. Our study is the first to demonstrate a significant inverse relationship between LVEF derived from gated SPECT and plasma cTnT on CCU discharge of post-AMI patients. We repeated LVEF estimate about three months after the onset of AMI because this parameter can be affected during the acute phase by a combination of myocardial necrosis, ischemia, periinfarction edema, and stunned myocardium (31). LV function and volumes may therefore not always represent true values in the acute phase after AMI, even if to acquire gated SPECT images at rest, as done in our study, may preserve from artifacts (22). The increase of the overall accuracy of cTnT in predicting LV function, when estimated three months after AMI, reinforces however our results.

In conclusion, the present study shows a clear relationship for cTnT on CCU discharge and SPECT parameters of infarct size and LV function in patients with a first AMI. Thus, a single measurement of plasma cTnT concentrations on the day of CCU discharge after AMI, regardless of the kinetic of marker appearance in blood, can be used as a convenient and cost-effective, noninvasive estimate of infarct size and for the assessment of LV function in routine clinical setting, revealing a similar reliability as peak CK-MB measurement (requiring however repetitive sampling) or nuclear imaging (not available in all patients in the acute phase of AMI and too expensive to be routinely used).

References

1. Sobel BE, Bresnahan GF, Shell WE, et al. (1972). Estimation of infarct size in man and its relation to prognosis. Circulation 46:640–648.
2. Vassanelli C, Menegatti G, Nidasio GP, et al. (1987). Comparison of different pharmacological interventions on enzymatic parameters during acute myocardial infarction. Clin Biochem 20:441–447.
3. Christenson RH, Vollmer RT, Ohman EM, et al. (2000). Relation of temporal creatine kinase-MB release and outcome after thrombolytic therapy for acute myocardial infarction. Am J Cardiol 85: 543–547.
4. HÖrder M, Hyltoft Petersen P, Thygesen K, et al. (1981). Plasma enzymes in myocardial infarction. An appraisal of quantitative, clinical and pathophysiological information. Scand J Clin Lab Invest 41:41–47.
5. Holman BL, Goldhaber SZ, Kirsch CM, et al. (1982). Measurement of infarct size using single photon emission computed tomography and technetium 99m pyrophosphate: A description of the method and comparison with patients prognosis. Am J Cardiol 50:503–511.
6. Kaul S (1998). Assessing the myocardium after attempted reperfusion. Should we bother? Circulation 98:625–627.
7. Grande P, Fischer Hansen B, Christiansen C, et al. (1982). Estimation of acute myocardial infarct size in man by serum CK-MB measurements. Circulation 65:756–764.
8. Hackel DB, Reimer KA, Ideker RE, et al. (1984). Comparison of enzymatic and anatomic estimates of myocardial infarct size in man. Circulation 70:824–835.
9. Grande P, Christiansen C, Alstrup K (1983). Comparison of ASAT, CK, CK-MB, and LD for the estimation of acute myocardial infarct size in man. Clin Chim Acta 128:329–335.
10. Burlina A, Rizzotti P, Plebani M, et al. (1984). CPK and CPK-MB in the early diagnosis of acute myocardial infarction and prediction of infarcted area. Clin Biochem 17:356–361.
11. Al-Saady NM, Camm AJ (1998). New soluble markers for assessment of infarct size. In: Kaski JC, Holt DW, eds. Myocardial damage. Early detection by novel biochemical markers. Kluwer Academic Publishers: Dordrecht, The Netherlands;137–148.
12. Katus HA, Remppis A, Scheffold T, et al. (1991). Intracellular compartmentation of cardiac troponin T and its release kinetics in patients with reperfused and nonreperfused myocardial infarction. Am J Cardiol 67:1360–1367.
13. Voss EM, Sharkey SW, Gernert AE, et al. (1995). Human and canine cardiac troponin T and creatine kinase-MB distribution in normal and diseases myocardium. Arch Pathol Lab Med 119:799–806.

14. Ricchiuti V, Sharkey SW, Murakami MM, et al. (1998). Cardiac troponin I and T alterations in dog hearts with myocardial infarction. Correlation with infarct size. Am J Clin Pathol 110:241–247.
15. Remppis A, Ehlermann P, Giannitsis E, et al. (2000). Cardiac troponin T levels at 96 hours reflect myocardial infarct size: A pathoanatomical study. Cardiology 93:249–253.
16. Hammerer-Lercher A, Metzler B, Mair J, et al. (2001). Cardiac troponin T closely correlates with infarct size in a murine model of acute myocardial infarction. Eur Heart J 22(Abstract Suppl):674.
17. Wagner I, Mair J, Fridrich L, et al. (1993). Cardiac troponin T release in acute myocardial infarction is associated with scintigraphic estimates of myocardial scar. Coron Artery Dis 4:537–544.
18. Tanaka H, Abe S, Yamashita T, et al. (1997). Serum levels of cardiac troponin I and troponin T in estimating myocardial infarct size soon after reperfusion. Coron Artery Dis 8:433–439.
19. Hallermayer K, Klenner D, Vogel R (1999). Use of recombinant human cardiac troponin T for standardization of third generation troponin T methods. Scand J Clin Lab Invest 59 (suppl 230):128–131.
20. Alpert J, Thygesen K, et al. for the Joint European Society of Cardiology/American College of Cardiology Committee (2000). Myocardial infarction redefined-A consensus document of the Joint European Society of Cardiology/American College of Cardiology Committee for the Redefinition of Myocardial Infarction. J Am Coll Cardiol 36:959–969.
21. Panteghini M, Gerhardt W, Apple FS, et al. (2001). Quality specifications for cardiac troponin assays. International Federation of Clinical Chemistry and Laboratory Medicine (IFCC) Scientific Division – Committee on Standardization of Markers of Cardiac Damage. Clin Chem Lab Med 39:174–178.
22. Bavelaar-Croon CDL, Pauwels EKJ, van der Wall EE (2001). Gated single-photon emission computed tomographic myocardial imaging: A new tool in clinical cardiology. Am Heart J 141:383–390.
23. The Multicenter Posinifarction Research Group (1983). Risk stratification and survival after myocardial infarction. N Engl J Med 309:331–336.
24. Kroll D, Farah W, McKendall GR, et al. (2001). Prognostic value of stress-gated Tc-99m sestamibi SPECT after acute myocardial infarction. Am J Cardiol 87:381–386.
25. Swets JA (1988). Measuring the accuracy of diagnostic systems. Science 240:1285–1293.
26. Wu AHB, Apple FS, Gibler WB, et al. (1999). National Academy of Clinical Biochemistry Standards of Laboratory Practice: Recommendations for the use of cardiac markers in coronary artery diseases. Clin Chem 45:1104–1121.
27. Mair J, Wagner I, Morass B, et al. (1995). Cardiac troponin I release correlates with myocardial infarction size. Eur J Clin Chem Clin Biochem 33;869–872.
28. Kragten JA, Hermens WT, van Dieijen-Visser MP (1996). Cardiac troponin T release into plasma after acute myocardial infarction: only fractional recovery compared with enzymes. Ann Clin Biochem 33:314–323.
29. Rao ACR, Collinson PO, Canepa-Anson R, et al. (1998). Troponin T measurement after myocardial infarction can identify left ventricular ejection of less than 40%. Heart 80:223–225.
30. Kanna M, Nonogi H, Sumida H, et al. (2001). Usefulness of serum troponin T levels on day three or four in predicting survival after myocardial infarction. Am J Cardiol 87:294–297.
31. Braunwald E, Kloner RA (1982). The stunned myocardium: prolonged, postischemic ventricular dysfunction. Circulation 66:1146–1149.

National Winner

Soluble Adhesion Molecules In Acute Stroke

A. M. Simundic, V. Basic, E. Topic, V. Demarin, N. Vrkic, B. Kunovic, M. Stefanovic, A. Begonja

Clinical Institute of Chemistry; Department of Molecular Diagnostics: University Hospital "SESTRE MILOSRDNICE": Zagreb, CROATIA

Abstract

Introduction

Cell adhesion molecules (CAM) are cell surface proteins that mediate cell-cell interactions and interactions of cells to certain extracellular matrix elements. A number of authors have reported elevated levels of soluble CAMs, as a result of cell activation, in subjects with a variety of pathological conditions. The upregulation of some adhesion molecules is found in acute stroke. The aim of this study was to assess plasma levels of sICAM-1, sVCAM-1, sE-selectin and sL-selectin in acute stroke and to investigate a relationship of CAMs with some stroke risk factors.

Methods

A total of 64 subjects admitted within 24 hours after onset of symptoms with acute ischemic stroke were included in the study. Diagnosis was established by history, neurological examination and cerebral CT scans. Demographic characteristics and risk factor profiles were collected for each patient. 77 healthy volunteers served as controls. Concentration of soluble adhesion molecules were determined with quantitative sandwich enzyme immunoassay method

Results

sICAM-1, sVCAM-1, sE-selectin levels were higher in patients with sL-selectin being higher in controls. Differences were statistically significant. sL-selectin inversely correlated with patient age. In controls sICAM-1 and sVCAM-1 tended to increase with advanced age, whereas sE-selectin levels were greater in men and sL-selectin in women. sL-selectin levels were higher in female patients and diabetics. Difference between CAM levels in regards to the severity of atherosclerotic changes in carotid vasculature was not found. Furthermore, mean CAM levels did not differ between smokers and non-smokers, hypertensive patients and those with normal blood pressure, hypercholesterolemic patients and those with normal blood cholesterol levels, and in patients with and without presence of infection. sICAM-1 and sL-selectin plasma levels correlated with blood glucose concentration in patients. Plasma levels of soluble CAMs correlated with other markers of inflammation, i.e. blood sedimentation rate, total leukocyte count and CRP concentration. ROC analysis showed that sICAM-1 has highest discriminating power in differentiating between acute stroke patients and healthy controls.

Conclusions

Elevated levels of sICAM-1, sVCAM-1 and sE-selectin reflect the activation of endothelial cells and leukocytes at the site of ischemic lesion. sL-selectin levels decrease in acute stroke probably a result of the activation of another counterreceptor for sL-selectin, needed for coupling of sL-selectins. Further studies should clarify the possible effect of administration of antibodies against adhesion molecules on ischemic cell damage after transient or permanent cerebral artery occlusion in humans.

NEPHROLOGY

National Winner

Monitoring Of The Renal Functions During Continuous Renal Replacement Therapy – The Application Of The Analysis Of Cystatin C And Natriuretic Peptides

M. Balik[1], A. Jabor[2], A. Hendl[2], M. Koláø[2], M. Pavlisová[2], D. Brestan[2]

[1] Dept. Anaesth and Intens.Care, University Hospital Vinohrady, Prague, CZECHIA
[2] Dept. Clinical Biochemistry, Hospital Kladno, CZECHIA
[3] Dept.of Kinanthropology, Charles University, Prague, CZECHIA

Abstract

Introduction

Continuous renal replacement therapy (CRRT) has become a routine therapeutic tool in an ICU over the last 15 years. CRRT enables better renal protection than intermittent dialysis with a consequent favorable impact on the outcome. The sensitive marker of glomerular filtration is cystatin C (cysC). It is a nonglycosylated basic protein produced at a constant rate by all nucleated cells. It is freely filtered by the renal glomeruli and catabolized in tubuli. No secretion or re-uptake in tubuli has been described. The serum concentration is independent of age, gender and muscle mass. Its molecular weight is 12500 Da and therefore cysC is classified as middle molecule which is eliminated predominantly by hemofiltration and possibly adsorption by the filter. There is little data about insignificant elimination of cysC by various filters in intermittent dialysis. CysC may be used as a marker of removal rate of low molecular weight protein on high flux membranes. No such data concerning CRRT has yet been published yet. The question is thus raised as to whether cysC can be used as a marker of residual glomerular filtration in patients on CRRT.

In these studies we assume that residual renal functions can be monitored by measuring the levels of cysC, ANP and BNP unless there are significant clearances on the filter. Monitoring of residual renal functions could have an impact on the renal protective regime. It could possibly influence even the choice of the mode of CRRT because of the different pattern of protein elimination in various modes of CRRT.

Methods

We conducted a prospective observational study using mechanically ventilated patients treated with early continuous venovenous hemodiafiltration (CVVHDF). The levels of ANP, BNP and cysC were measured before and during 48 hours of CVVHDF. Samples were drawn both from the ports proximal and distal to the filter. ANP levels (normal < 14 pmol/L) and BNP levels (normal < 5.3 pmol/L) were analysed in 13 patients. CysC levels (normal < 0.99 mg/L) were measured in 16 patients. Arteriovenous concentration differences (A-Vdiff.) were calculated. According to the configuration of the CVVHDF, a value greater than –6.9% reflects sieving, adsorption or both. Furosemide was reduced to 1.5 mg/kg. day after the commencing of CVVHDF. Left ventricular dysfunction (LVD) was defined as LV ejection fraction below 40%. Patients were divided according to the daily diuresis (Vu) after 48h of treatment into groups with Vu < 3000 ml/24h and groups which retained Vu > 3000 ml/24h. A control groups consisted of 10 patients exposed to abdominal surgery for the natriuretic peptide study and of 65 similar patients for the cysC study.

Results

The average AVdiff (%) of ANP was –3.68+/–48.72 and of BNP was –4.04+/–23.68. Significant correlations were revealed for ANP and Vu (r = –0.40, p<0.02) and for BNP and Vu (r=–0.43, p<0.007). Patients with increasing diuresis on CVVHDF (n=8) had significantly lower levels of both ANP (8.96+/–13.19 pmol/L) and BNP (100.85+/–159.31 pmol/L) than the patients with decreasing diuresis (n=5) (26.83+/–13.94 pmol/l (p<0.004) for ANP, resp. 356.22+/–298.81 pmol/L (p<0.01) for BNP). The levels of both peptides were grossly elevated in comparison to controls and were predictive of survival. The differences between cardiac and non-cardiac patients were not significant either for ANP or for BNP. Average AVdiff (%) of cysC was +5.73+/–15.57. Patients with increasing diuresis on CVVHDF (n=7) had significantly lower levels of cysC (2.52+/–1.59 mg/l) than patients with decreasing diuresis (n=9) (3.44+/–0.69 mg/L, p<0.04). A significant correlation between cysC and Vu was found, in particular for the cysC levels below 4.0 mg/l (r=–0.76 (p<0.002)). The levels of cysC predicted survival.

Conclusions

The elimination of cysC, ANP and BNP by the CVVHDF is negligible. The levels of cysC and natriuretic peptides are inversely related to Vu. Whether cysC could be used as an indicator of successful weaning from CVVHDF needs to be confirmed by further study. The levels of cysC, ANP and BNP predict survival of patients treated with CVVHDF. ANP and BNP levels did not correlate with LVD, which may be caused by their elevation due to renal failure.

HAEMATOLOGY – HAEMOSTATIS

National Winners

Serum Levels Of Soluble Transferrin Receptors (STFR) Correlate Better With Severity Of Disease Than With Iron Stores In Patients With Malignant Lymphomas

J. Bjerner, L. M. Amlie, L. S. Rusten, E. Jakobsen

Central Laboratory, Norwegian Radium Hospital, Montebello, N-0310 Oslo, NORWAY

Abstract

Introduction

Serum sTfR levels in serum may be useful in differentiating between Iron Deficiency Anemia (IDA) and Anemia of Chronic Disease (ACD). However, there is both theoretical and clinical evidence for elevated sTfR levels in patients with various hematological malignancies.

Methods

Routine bone marrow aspirations were performed in 82 patients with malignant lymphomas (63 with NHL and 19 with Hodgkin's disease). Smears were stained for evaluation of iron stores and graded. Patients were also given a disease score based on bone marrow morphology, ESR and LDH.

Results

Serum levels of sTfR correlated better with disease score (partial r_s controlled for iron stores was 0.51 (0.39–0.65) $p < 0.001$) than with iron stores (partial r_s controlled for disease score was –0.25 (–0.44 – –0.03) $p = 0.027$).

Conclusions

This study shows elevated levels of sTfR in patients with malignant lymphomas without any signs of IDA. The diagnosis of IDA should not be established upon sTfR alone in this group of patients.

The Functional Activity Of Platelets In Surgery Patients With Artificial Cardiac Valve

T. Lobachevskaya, T. Vavilova, M. Kadinskaya, D. Polezhaev

The Pavlov's Medical University, St. Petersburg, RUSSIA

Abstract

Introduction

Thromboembolic complications remain as one of the main problems in patients with mechanical heart valves. The aim of this investigation was to assess the thin, initial changes of functional activity of platelets in patients with ACV, to compare the new Laser method of platelet activity value with traditional approach in the investigation of vascular-thrombocytic hemostasis and also to assess the risk of chronic DIC development in the given group of patients.

Methods

Sixty eight patients in far-removed terms (1.5–2.5 years) after the operation în isolated prothestic of bycuspidal cardiac valve were examined in order to work out optimum methods of laboratory analysis of vascular-thrombocytic hemostasis and to assess the adequate of anticoagulation. All the patients had the heart failure I – II by NYHA and received oral anticoagulants.The patients were divided into two groups according INR. We used 3 methods of assessment of vascular-thrombocytic hemostasis, and the test on definition of D-dimer ("Roche") was included in the investigation.

Results

The value of functional activity of platelets by Laser method revealed significant disorders. The majority of patients in both groups (92%) had the high date of intravascular activity of platelets. The inducting aggregation by G.V.R.Born showed the differences between 1 and 2 groups of patients, particularly in induction 1,25 μg/mL and 0,625 μg/mL doses ADP. Patients from 2 group had disorders in coagulation system: the lower level of fibrinogen and positive reaction to D-dimer.

Conclusions

This data has shown that inadequate anticoagulation in patients with artificial cardiac valve (ACV) leads to the dangerous disorders in the system of vascular-thrombocytic hemostasis with marks of continuous disseminated intravascular coagulation syndrome (DIC). In addition, our data have shown that inadequate anticoagulation in patients with artificial cardiac valve (ACV) leads to the dangerous disorders in the system of vascular- thrombocytic hemostasis with marks of continuous disseminated intravascular coagulation syndrome (DIC).

Serum Oxidative State Following Thrombolysis Combined With ABCIXIMAB In Comparison To r-PA Or Streptokinase Alone

I. Maor[1], G. Slobodin[1], E. Goldhammer[2], S. Shnizer[1], T. Kagan[1], E. G. Abinader[2], A. Lanir[1]

Departments of Biochemistry[1] and Cardiology[2], Bnai Zion Medical Center, Faculty of Medicine[2], Technion, Haifa, ISRAEL

Abstract

Introduction

Increased oxidative state has been previously demonstrated in several trials of myocardial reperfusion using a single-agent thrombolytic therapy. Combination therapy with Abciximab, a platelet glycoprotein IIb/IIIa inhibitor and reduced-dose t-PA (tissue Plasminogen Activator) has been suggested to improve myocardial reperfusion. However, its effect on radical activity has not been studied yet.

Methods

In order to evaluate the effect of combined thrombolyic therapy on the oxidative stress in serum, 65 patients with acute infarction were treated with either recombinant t-PA (r-PA, n=20) alone or Abciximab combined with r-PA (n=25) or with Streptokinase (STK, n=20). Blood samples were collected before thrombolysis and 30 minutes, 1, 3 and 24 hours post thrombolysis and the oxidative state was determined in the serum samples by 3 different methods.

Results

The levels of serum lipid peroxides (PD) were significantly ($p<0.01$) increased by 45%, 49% and 60%, 30 minutes after treatment with either r-PA, Abciximab combined with r-PA or with STK respectively, followed by a time-dependent decrease in the PD levels. Twenty four hours after thrombolysis, PD values were 10% lower in the combined therapy, while in patients that received r-PA or STK alone, PD values in serum were 7% and 19% higher respectively then their initial values.

Similarly, thiobarbituric acid reactive substances (TBARS) were also increased in serum by 41%, 24% and 34% respectively following treatment, while 24 hours following treatment, TBARS levels were 9% lower in the combined therapy, 6% and 10% higher then initial values in r-PA and STK groups. Protein carbonyl concentrations were used as a marker of oxidized proteins in the serum. Their levels were significantly increased following the thrombolytic treatment, and remained elevated for several hours. Twenty four hours after thrombolysis, protein carbonyl levels were 15%, 16% and 10% lower in the combined treatment group, in r-PA or STK groups respectively in comparison to their initial values.

As activated neutrophils are a potential source of oxygen free radicals, we studied the effect of a thrombolytic agent and IIb/IIIa platelets antagonist on superoxide release by human neutrophils. Incubation of the activated cells with increasing concentrations of r-PA (0.01–0.06 U/ml) or with Abciximab (5–30 μg/mL) led to a significant dose-dependent reduction by up to 46% and 36% respectively in superoxide production by the neutrophils. When r-PA and Abciximab were both added to neutrophils (0.02 U/ml r-PA +5 μg/mL ABCIXIMAB), however, a significant ($p<0.01$) inhibition by up of 60% was observed.

Conclusions

Based on these results, we concluded that the thrombolytic treatment, and the combined therapy in particular reduces oxidative stress by inhibiting superoxide production by the neutrophils, and thus might potentially lead to less tissue reperfusion injury.

NEW TECHNOLOGY – METHODS

Finalists

A Rapid And Sensitive Immunoassay For Determination Of S-100 Protein In A Point-Of-Care Setting

S. Eriksson,[1] L. Dean,[2] K. Pettersson[1]

[1] Department of Biotechnology, University of Turku, FINLAND
[2] School of Biomedical and Life Sciences, University of Surrey, Guildford, UK

Abstract

Introduction

The S-100 family of proteins are acidic calcium-binding proteins comprising 19 members. S-100B is most abundant in glial cells in the brain and it forms either homodimers or heterodimers together with S-100A1. Protein S-100B has, in addition to its use in malignant melanoma and brain trauma, been proposed as a marker of brain damage in cardiac arrest patients. An increase in S-100B levels reflects the degree of hypoxic brain damage and predicts the short-term outcome. However, existing assays lack ease of use and usually require several hours to perform. The aim of this work was to establish a rapid and sensitive immunoassay for measurement of S-100B, which could be used in a near-patient environment.

Methods

Seven commercially available monoclonal antibodies (CanAg Diagnostics, Sweden, and HyTest, Finland) were tested. The final antibody pair was selected with rapid kinetics, high sensitivity and good correlation with the Sangtec 100 assay as the main criteria. S-100 protein purified from human brain consisting of S-100BB and S-100A1B (HyTest, Finland) was used for calibration. Serum, heparin plasma or whole blood can be analysed with the assay, which is based on an all-in-one dry reagent concept (1). All the analyte-specific reagents are built into a single streptavidin coated microtiter well in a dry stable form. The capture antibody is biotinylated and the tracer antibody is labelled with a highly stable, inherently fluorescent europium chelate that can be detected by time-resolved fluorometry directly from the surface without a separate signal development step.

Results

The sample incubation step is only 15 minutes, which gives a total turn-around time of less than 20 minutes. The measuring range is between 0.1 and 62.5 µg/L, with a detection limit lower than 0.05 µg/L using 20 µL of sample. The correlation with the Sangtec 100 assay was excellent ($r=0.99, n=20$) in a preliminary evaluation.

Conclusions

We were able to develop a sensitive and rapid assay for the measurement of S-100B, which is suitable for simple, automated processing of single specimens in a point-of-care setting. The short turn-around time of the assay should speed up the diagnosis and facilitate more rapid and effective treatment of critical care patients. The developed concept allows near-patient testing to be performed while preserving state-of-art central laboratory performance characteristics. The clinical value of the rapid S-100 assay is still not fully ascertained.

Reference

1. Lövgren T, Meriö L, Mitrunen K et al. One-step all-in-one dry reagent immunoassays with fluorescent europium chelate label and time-resolved fluorometry. Clin Chem 1996; 42:1196–1201.

Introduction

The S100 protein family consists of 19 members that are differentially expressed in a large number of cell types. The acidic, calcium binding S100 proteins were discovered in 1965 as a brain protein fraction (1) which later was shown to consist of two closely related molecules S100A1 and S100B (previously known as S100a and S100b) (2). These two monomers form homo- or heterodimers, designed S100BB, S100A1B and S100A1A1. In mammals, S100BB is most abundant in glial and Schwann cells while S100A1B is present in glial cells. S100A1A1 is present in striated muscles, heart and kidney. Since S100B concentrations in the blood of a normal healthy population are very low, measurement of S100B can be used as a sensitive and specific marker for central nervous system dysfunction. Elevated concentrations of S100B have been detected in patients with minor head injury (3), stroke (4, 5), cardiac arrest (6) and recently also in Creutzfeld-Jacob disease (7). Serum S100B has also been used as a marker of cerebral damage during cardiac surgery (8) although a recent report claims that the increase in S100B arises from extracerebral sources of contamination (9). S100B is also used for clinical staging and monitoring of malignant melanoma (10) and as well as a prognostic marker (11).

Elevated S100B concentrations in cerebrospinal fluid have been found in the earlier stages of Alzheimer's disease (12) and also in serum of schizophrenic patients (13).

Existing S100 assays lack ease of use and usually take several hours to perform. Rapid, sensitive point-of-care assays could be very useful for managing critically ill patients and for assessing the severity of head trauma. One-step all-in-one immunoassays that use time-resolved fluorescence for detection have previously been reported for cardiac markers (14) and model assays have also been developed for human chorionic gonadotropon, a-fetoprotein and progesterone (15). The all-in-one immunoassays are performed in microtitration wells containing all assay-specific components in a stable dry form. Addition of the sample and a common assay buffer starts the reaction, which is completed in 15 min or less. The aim of this work was to establish a rapid and sensitive point-of-care assay for the measurement of S100B in whole blood, serum and plasma.

Materials and Methods

Immunoreagents

Four monoclonal antibodies (coded C1, C2, C3 and C4) were from CanAg Diagnostics, Gothenburg, Sweden and three monoclonal antibodies (coded H1, H2 and H3) were from HyTest Ltd, Turku, Finland. Human S100BB protein purified from human brain was from HyTest Ltd and it was used for standardisation. Human S100 consisting of a mixture of S100BB and S100A1B was also form HyTest Ltd. Bovine S100AA, S100A1B and S100BB were purchased from Affiniti Research Products Ltd, Exeter, United Kingdom and used for testing the specificity of the assay. Standards were prepared in a buffer containing 7.5% bovine serum albumin, 50 mmol/L Tris-HCl pH 7.75, 15 mmol/L NaCl, 0.5 g/L NaN_3 and 2.5 mmol/L $CaCl_2$.

Labelling with lanthanide chelates and biotinylation

The europium chelate used for labelling of the detection antibodies was kindly provided by M.Sc. Jaana Rosenberg (Department of Bio-organic Chemistry, University of Turku). The chelate was a europium chelate of 2,2',2",2'"-{[2-(4-Isothiocyanatophenyl)ethylimino]bis(methylene)bis{4-{[4-(a-galactopyranoxy) phenyl]ethynyl}pyridine-2,6-diyl}bis(methylenenitrilo)}tetrakis(acetic acid)}. The labelling of antibodies was performed in 10 mM sodium borate buffer pH 8.6 with a 100-fold molar excess of chelate at room temperature over night. The labelled antibody was separated from excess free label on a Superdex 200 HR 10/30 gel filtration column equilibrated and run with 50 mmol/L Tris-HCl pH 7.75, 15 mmol/L NaCl, 0.5 g/L NaN_3 at 15 mL/h and 0.5-mL fractions were collected. The fractions containing labeled protein were pooled, the protein concentration was determined with Bradford protein assay and the degree of labelling was determined using a europium calibration solution. Bovine serum albumin was added to a final concentration of 1 g/L and the solution was filtered through a 0.22 μm pore size filter and stored at +4°C until use.

For the biotinylation of antibodies biotin-isothiocyanate (J. Rosenberg) was used. The antibody was biotinylated with a 30-fold molar excess of biotinylation reagent in 50 mM carbonate buffer pH 9.8 at room temperature for 4 h. The biotinylated antibody was separated from free biotinylation reagent by passing the reaction twice through disposable gelfiltration columns. Bovine serum albumin was added to a final concentration of 1 g/L and the solution was filtered through a 0.22 μm pore size filter and stored at +4°C until use.

Preparation of dry reagent microtitration single wells

Streptavidin coated single wells (Innotrac Diagnostics Oy, Turku, Finland) were used for immobilisation of capture antibody. 400 ng of biotinylated antibody in Assay Buffer (PerkinElmer Life Sciences Wallac, Turku, Finland) was immobilised by incubating for one hour at 35°C without shaking. The wells were then washed twice with Delfia Wash Buffer (PerkinElmer Wallac) with a modified plate washer (Delfia Platewash 1296-096, PerkinElmer Wallac). 40 μl of an insulating layer (15) supplemented with 1.5 mmol/l $CaCl_2$ was added to each well. The wells were dried over night at 35°C and 5% relative humidity. The europium labelled tracer antibody (100 ng/well) was dispensed on top of the insulating layer in a total volume of 1 μl using an in-house automatic tracer dispenser. The dispensed solution was dried immediately by blowing air into the well. The ready dry reagent wells were packed into pens and stored at room temperature in a sealed package with desiccant.

Immunoassay procedures

The Innotrac Aio! Immunoanalyzer (Innotrac Diagnostics) was used to perform the assays. The machine added 20 μl of the standards or samples to the wells, followed by 10 μl of Aio buffer (Innotrac Diagnostics), and this started the reaction. The wells were incubated for 15 min at 36°C, washed six times and dried. The instrument measured the time-resolved europium fluorescence directly from the dried well.

Samples

Serum, plasma and whole blood samples with heparin as anticoagulant were taken from apparently healthy volunteers at the Department of Biotechnology, University of Turku. Additional serum samples were analysed with the LIAISON® Sangtec®100 assay (AB Sangtec Medical, Bromma, Sweden) by Ph.D. Henrik Alfthan, Department of Clinical Chemistry, Helsinki University Central Hospital.

Results

Selection of antibody pair

All 49 combinations of capture and tracer antibodies were tested in sandwich assays. The combinations that gave the highest specific counts taking into account the labelling degree were further evaluated with kinetic experiments in order to find a pair that was close to equilibrium after only 15 minutes of incubation. The specific counts divided by the labelling degree of the tracer antibody is shown in Figure 1 with C3 as capture antibody and different tracer antibodies. C3 was selected as the capture antibody and H2 as the tracer antibody, due to their high specific signals, rapid kinetics and good correlation with the Sangtec 100 assay when 20 serum samples were measured (data not shown).

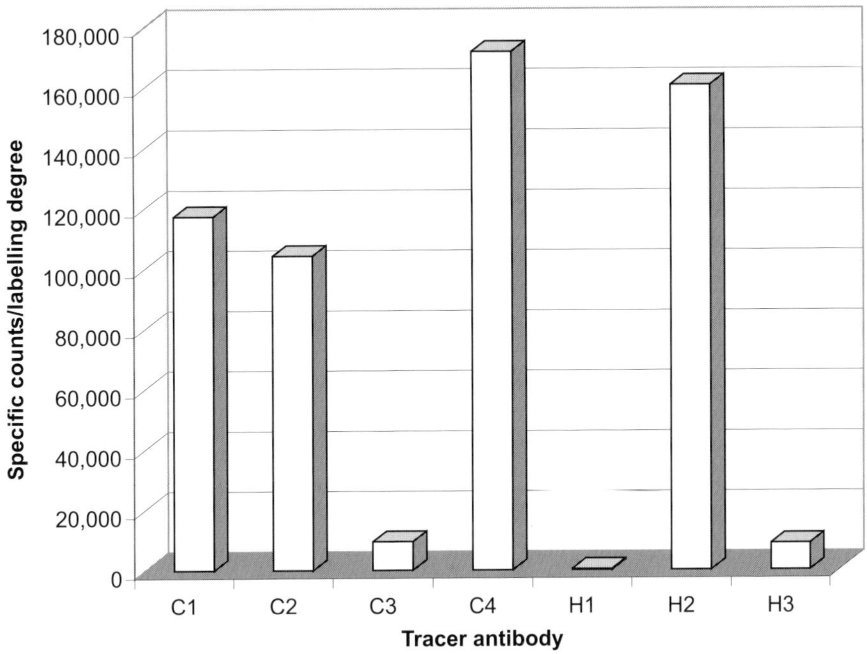

Figure 1. Specific signals with C3 as capture antibody and different tracer antibodies. The differences in labelling degrees were corrected by dividing the specific signal with the labelling degree of the antibody.

Calibration curve

A typical calibration curve based on ten assays performed with standards in duplicate is shown in Figure 2. The standard curve is stored in the instrument and new calibration is needed only when a new batch of reagents is taken into use. No high dose hook was seen at a S100BB concentration of 650 µg/L, even if the standard curve is no longer linear above 62.5 µg/L. The analytical detection limit of the S100B assay calculated as the mean value of the blank + 3 standard deviations was 0.017 µg/L.

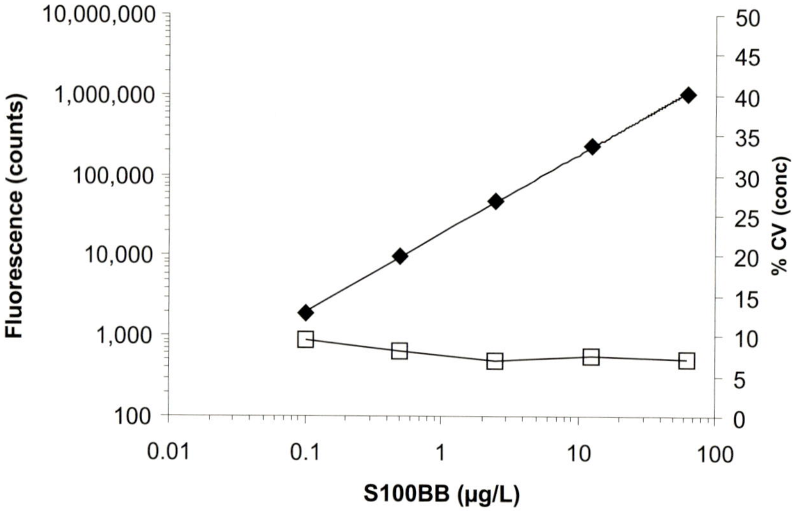

Figure 2. Calibration curve (◆) and inter-assay precision profile (□) based on mean signals from 10 separate runs with standards measured in duplicate.

Between-assay variation

The between-assay variation was measured by repeated measurements of standards or samples in duplicate for five days with two separate runs each day. The coefficient of variation (CV) for the counts of the blank was 10.9%, the CV for the other standards based on calculated concentration are shown in Figure 2 (range 6.8–9.4%). The CV for a serum sample containing 0.058 µg/L S100B was 5.2%, for a heparin plasma sample with 0.338 µg/L S100B the CV was 7.9% and for a serum sample spiked with S100BB to a concentration of 2.037 µg/L the CV was 5.4%.

Sample matrix

The effect of the sample matrix was investigated by comparing S100B concentrations in serum, heparin plasma and heparin whole blood samples taken from 20 apparently healthy volunteers. The mean S100B concentration in serum was 0.087 µg/L (median 0.075, range 0.029–0.207) in heparin plasma 0.125 µg/L (median

0.098, range 0.029–0.341) and in whole blood without hematocrit correction 0.111 µg/L (median 0.074, range 0.025–0.384). The values in heparin plasma were 97–249% (mean 141%, median 130%) of the serum values, the values in whole blood were 49–218% of the serum values (mean 125%, median 125%), and 37–130% of the heparin plasma values (mean 88%, median 89%). The results are shown in Figure 3A.

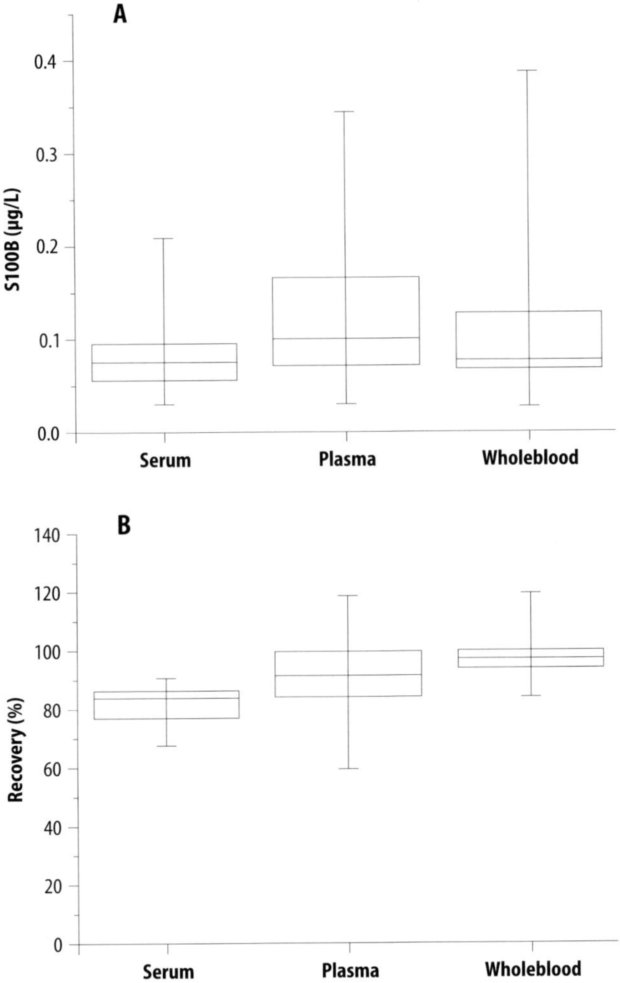

Figure 3. Box-whisker plots show the S100B concentrations in different sample matrices from 20 volunteers (A) and the recovery of human S100BB (2.5 µg/L) in the same sample matrices (B). The horizontal line depicts the median concentration, the upper and lower edges of box the 25th and 75th percentiles and the lines extending above and below the box the measured minimum and maximum values.

Analytical recovery

The analytical recovery was tested by adding human S100BB to serum, heparin plasma or whole blood samples (n=20) to a concentration of 2.5 μg/L. The average recovery in serum was 82% (median 83%, range 68–91%) in heparin plasma 91% (median 90%, range 59–118%) and in whole blood 97% (median 96%, range 83–119%). The results are shown in Figure 3B.

Effect of dilution

To study the effect of dilution, serum, heparin plasma and whole blood samples were diluted in the buffer used for dilution of standards or in serum or plasma with low S100B concentration. The measured results were compared with the calculated values. Dilution of serum and heparin plasma gave values close to the expected, but dilution of whole blood gave higher values than expected as shown in Figure 4. The linearity of dilution of S100BB standard in serum and plasma was tested by adding different amounts of S100BB to samples to give concentrations between 0.02 μg/L and 62.5 μg/L. The linearity was good over the whole range in serum, and in plasma only the lowest concentration, 0.02 μg/L, was not quite in the linear range as shown in Figure 5.

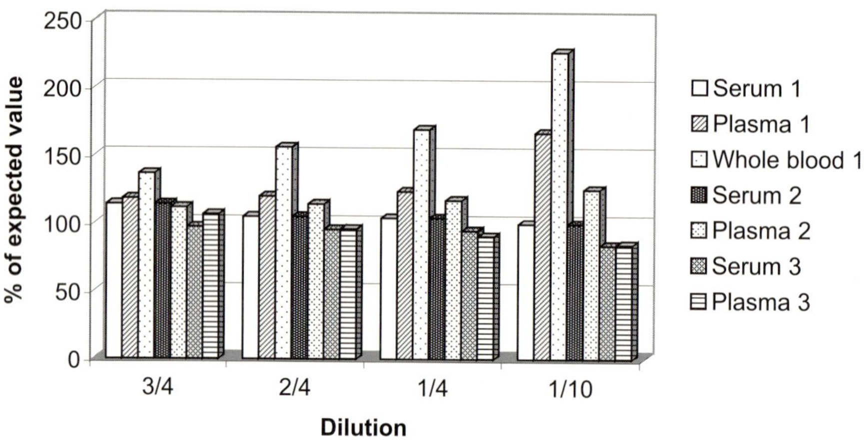

Figure 4. Dilution of serum, heparin plasma and whole blood in buffer used for dilution of standards (numbers 1 and 2) or in another serum or plasma sample with low concentration (number 3).

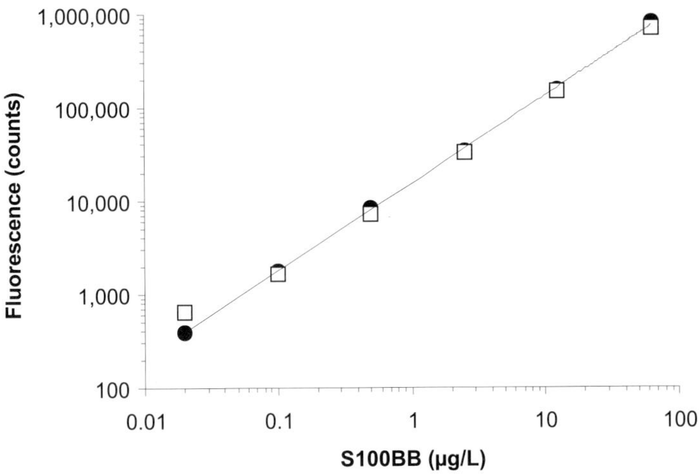

Figure 5. Linearity of diluting standard S100BB in serum (l) and in plasma (•). The counts from the sample without any addition were subtracted. Addition of 0.02 µg/L S100BB can be reliably measured.

Comparison with commercial assay

Eighty two serum samples analysed with the LIAISON Sangtec 100 were also measured with the new S100B assay. The correlation between the two assays was good with an *r*-value of 0.967, a slope of 1.021 and a y-intercept of –0.020 as shown in Figure 6.

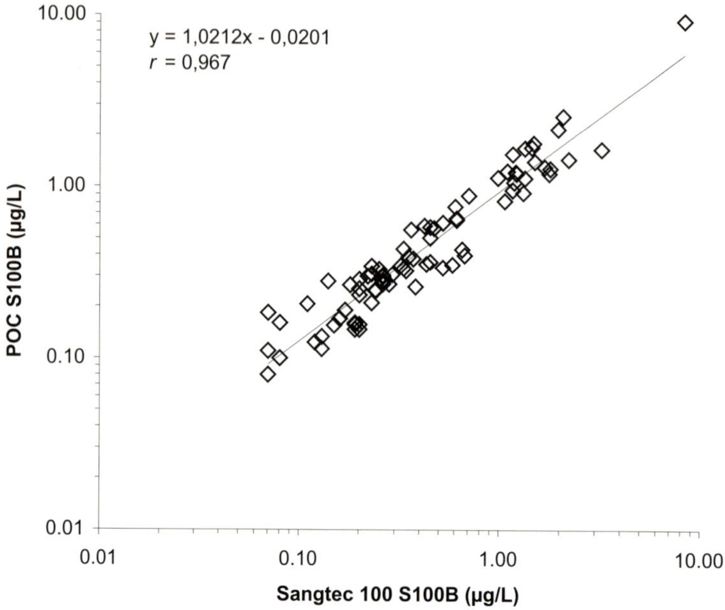

Figure 6. Linear regression analysis of the results of S100B measurement of 82 serum samples with the LIAISON Sangtec 100 assay (on the *x* axis) and with the new POC S100 assay (on the *y* axis). The equation of the line of regression and the correlation coefficient are indicated in the figure.

Cross-reactivity with S100 isoforms

The cross-reactivity with bovine S100A1A1, S100A1B and S100BB was evaluated by diluting the protein in the same buffer as used for the standards. The cross-reactivity with S100A1A1 was 0.97% at 62.5 µg/L. The signal of bovine S100BB was 2.7 times higher than that of human S100BB at 62.5 µg/L. The signal obtained with bovine S100A1B was only slightly lower than with bovine S100BB. Human S100 protein consisting of a mixture of A1B and BB (ratio not known) gave about 82% of the human S100BB signal. The binding curves for the different isoforms are shown in Figure 7. The difference in signals from bovine and human S100BB is probably due to differences in determining the protein concentration by the two producers, and we directly used the concentration reported by the manufacturer.

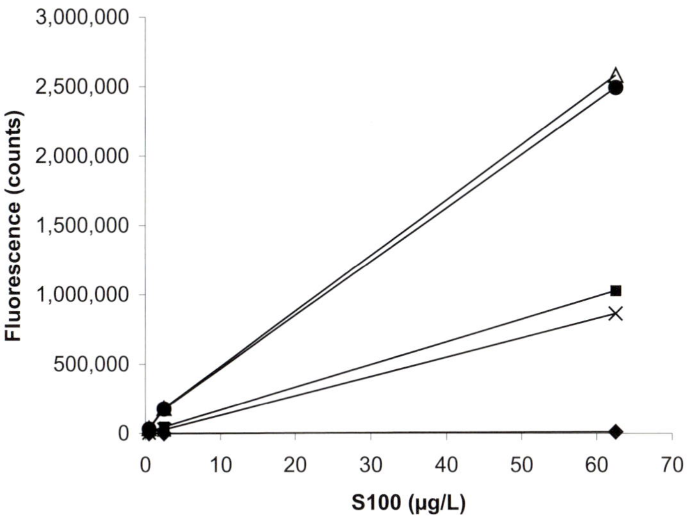

Figure 7. Binding curves for the S100B assay with S100 isoforms, bovine BB (D), bovine A1B (l), bovine AA (u), human BB (n) and a mixture of human A1B and BB(´).

Stability of S100 in different matrices

Aliquots of serum, heparin plasma and whole blood as such or spiked with 2.5 µg/L human S100BB were stored for 4 days at room temperature or at +4°C. The stability of endogenous S100B in serum was good, no change in activity could be seen after four days of storage. In heparin plasma the signal was slightly reduced but it was still more than 80% of the original after 4 days of storage at both temperatures. The stability of standard S100BB was poorer than that of the endogenous S100BB. The storage of whole blood is not recommended since one of the whole blood samples gave highly increased signals (non-specific) after storage (data not shown). The spiked whole blood sample also showed some increase in signals up to 120% of the original after 4 days of storage at +4°C. The stability of serum and heparin plasma was a bit better at +4°C than at room temperature. Serum and heparin samples can be stored for several days at +4°C (or even at room temperature), but the storage of whole blood is not recommended.

S100B concentration in samples with high CRP concentration

Based on the finding that some of the volunteers had slightly increased S100B values compared to the average and that most of these volunteers reported having a cold or some other infection, serum samples with high C-reactive protein (CRP) concentrations were also analysed with the S100B assay. Twenty samples with CRP concentrations ranging from 71–349 mg/L were measured with the S100B assay.

No significant correlation could be found between CRP and S100B concentrations (r=0.377, P=0.101). In seven samples the S100B was below 0.1 µg/L, seven samples were between 0.1 and 0.2 µg/L, and six samples had concentrations higher than 0.2 µg/L. The highest S100B value, 0.974 µg/L was found in a sample with a CRP concentration of 329 mg/L. Of the 20 volunteers, 15 had serum S100B values below 0.1 µg/L, four had values between 0.1 and 0.2 µg/L and one had a value of 0.207 µg/L. The mean S100B value in samples with high CRP concentrations was 0.206 µg/L, compared to 0.087 µg/L in the samples from the volunteers, with a statistically significant difference between the means (P=0.029). There are reports of association between high serum levels of S100B and cytokine inflammatory mediators (16) and S100 protein members are known to have a role in the regulation of inflammation (17). In order to confirm that infections cause elevated S100B values more samples with clinical information must be tested.

Conclusions

We have technically validated a new, rapid POC assay for measuring S100B in serum, plasma and whole blood. The low detection limit of the assay (0.017 µg/L) allowed reliable measurement of all 20 samples tested from healthy volunteers. The between-assay variation was below 10% and the measuring range was linear up to 62.5 µg/L. The analytical recovery of standard S100BB was with only a few exceptions good and dilution of serum and plasma presented no problems, but the dilution of whole blood did not quite give the expected results. Comparison to a commercial assay showed a good correlation between S100B results. The cross-reactivity with S100A1A1 is negligible and the signal of S100A1B is close to the signal of S100BB. Serum and plasma can be stored for several days without any change in S100B reactivity. Long-term (even overnight) storage of whole blood, however, is not recommended. This new assay should now be clinically validated with carefully selected patient material to establish the clinical value of the assay in different medical conditions.

The possibility to use whole blood for the analysis speeds up the analysis, since no time is required for the separation of plasma or serum. In the LIAISON Sangtec 100 assay it is only possible to use serum or cerebrospinal fluid as sample material. One optical immunoassay for detection of S100B in whole blood has previously been reported, but it uses a methanol-based extraction reagent in order to reduce the interference from whole blood in the assay (18). The detection limit of the optical assay in blood was 0.25 µg/L. The fact that whole blood without hematocrit correction gives values very close to those of heparin plasma might indicate that whole blood causes some interference resulting in a higher background level. The reason for the minor differences in results from serum, heparin plasma and whole blood is not known at the moment, but further investigations into this are necessary. One previous paper has reported that values in heparin plasma were 93–151% of the serum values (19). EDTA plasma was not tested in our study, since early tests showed that the signal obtained from S100 is dependent on the calcium concentration in the sample, and the values in EDTA plasma have been reported to be only 20–46% of the serum values (19). The limitation of our procedure that only whole blood and plasma with heparin as an anticoagulant can be used is not likely to be a problem.

The reference values reported for a healthy population varies greatly depending on the assay. With the LIAISON Sangtec 100 assay 95% of healthy men and women have S100B values below 0.15 μg/L in serum. One assay with a detection limit of 0.0125 μg/L reports a mean S100B value of 0.0067 μg/L with a 98th percentile of 0.021 μg/L (19). Another assay with a detection limit of 0.015 μg/L gives a reference value for S100B of 0.069±0.058 μg/L (20). The concentration of S100B in cerebrospinal fluid has been reported to be age- and sex-related with an increase with age (21) but in blood no significant relation has been found (22). The values of the 20 volunteers in this study are probably not representative for the total population, since the age distribution was skewed with the majority (n=15) of the volunteers in the age group of 21–30 years, three volunteers between 31–40 years and only two between 41–50 years. The highest S100B concentrations were actually found in the youngest age group. The number of volunteers was also much too low for any final conclusions to be made from this material. Based on the results from the correlation between the assays and the measured concentrations in healthy subjects, the new assay seem to have very similar characteristics when it comes to specificity and reference values as the Sangtec 100 assay. Further investigations are needed to confirm the possible relationship between inflammation and S100B.

The fact that increased S100 levels are found in a number of very different conditions, from brain trauma to malignant melanoma, and the recent report of high serum S100B levels in trauma patients without head injury (23) make interpretation of S100B levels very important. The result must always be interpreted in connection with the overall clinical status and other diagnostic procedures. The negative predictive value of S100B may however be of great importance to exclude brain tissue damage after trauma (23). Most of the reported assays for S100, as well as our new POC assay, measure the B-subunit of S100 dimers, which means that the S100 dimer must consist of at least one B-subunit in order to be detected and thus both S100BB and S100A1B will be detected by these assays. Recently there was a report of S100A1B and S100BB specific assays (24) that were used to possibly distinguish between S100 of cerebral and extracerebral origin (9). In that study however, both S100BB and S100A1B were detected from extracerebral sources.

We were able to develop a rapid and sensitive S100B assay that fulfils the requirements for POC assays and is suitable for simple, automated processing of single specimens. The developed concept allows near-patient testing to be performed while preserving state-of-the-art central laboratory performance characteristics. The short turn-around time and continuous availability of the assay should speed up the diagnosis and facilitate more rapid and effective treatment of critical care patients.

Acknowledgements

The antibodies used in this work were kindly supplied by CanAg Diagnostics, Sweden, and HyTest Ltd, Finland. The Innotrac Aio! instrument was provided by Innotrac Diagnostics Oy, Finland. Financial support was received from the National Technology Agency in Finland (TEKES).

We thank Ph.D. Henrik Alfthan for measuring the S100 samples and for his collaboration in this project. The skilful technical assistance of M.Sc. Eeva-Katri Kumpula and B.Sc. Mari Peltola is gratefully acknowledged. Mrs. Pirjo Laaksonen and Mrs. Sari Lindgren are thanked for taking the blood samples.

References

1. Moore BW (1965) A soluble protein characteristic of the nervous system. Biochem Biophys Res Commun 19:739–744
2. Isobe T, Okuyama T (1981) The amino-acid sequence of the alpha subunit in bovine brain S-100a protein. Eur J Biochem 116:79–86
3. Ingebrigtsen T, Romner B, Trumpy JH (1997) Management of minor head injury: the value of early computed tomography and serum protein S-100 measurements. J Clin Neuroscience 4:29–33
4. Abraha HD, Butterworth RJ, Bath PM, Wassif WS, Garthwaite J, Sherwood RA (1997) Serum S-100 protein, relationship to clinical outcome in acute stroke. Ann Clin Biochem 34:366–70
5. Wunderlich MT, Ebert AD, Kratz T, Goertler M, Jost S, Herrmann M (1999) Early neurobehavioral outcome after stroke is related to release of neurobiochemical markers of brain damage. Stroke 30:1190–5
6. Rosén H, Rosengren L, Herlitz J, Blomstrand C (1998) Increased serum levels of the S-100 protein are associated with hypoxic brain damage after cardiac arrest. Stroke 29:473–7
7. Otto M, Wiltfang J, Schütz E, et al (1998) Diagnosis of Creutzfeldt-Jakob disease by measurement of S100 protein in serum: prospective case-control study. BMJ 316:577–82
8. Shaaban Ali M, Harmer M, Vaughan R (2000) Serum S100 protein as a marker of cerebral damage during cardiac surgery. Br J Anaesth 85:287–98
9. Anderson RE, Hansson LO, Nilsson O, Liska J, Settergren G, Vaage J (2001) Increase in serum S100A1-B and S100BB during cardiac surgery arises from extracerebral sources. Ann Thorac Surg 71:1512–7
10. Guo HB, Stoffel-Wagner B, Bierwirth T, Mezger J, Klingmuller D (1995) Clinical significance of serum S100 in metastatic malignant melanoma. Eur J Cancer 31A:1898–902
11. von Schoultz E, Hansson LO, Djureen E, et al (1996) Prognostic value of serum analyses of S-100 beta protein in malignant melanoma. Melanoma Res 6:133–7
12. Peskind E, Griffin S, Akama K, Raskind M, van Eldik L (2001) Cerebrospinal fluid S100B is elevated in the earlier stages of Alzheimer's disease. Neurochem Int 39:409–413
13. Lara DR, Gama CS, Belmonte-de-Abreu P, et al (2001) Increased serum S100B protein in schizophrenia: a study in medication-free patients. J Psychiatr Res 35:11–4
14. Pettersson K, Katajamäki T, Irjala K, Leppänen V, Majamaa-Voltti K, Laitinen P (2000) Time-resolved fluorometry (TRF)-based immunoassay concept for rapid and quantitative determination of biochemical myocardial infarction markers from whole blood, serum and plasma. Luminescence 15:399–407
15. Lövgren T, Meriö L, Mitrunen K, et al (1996) One-step all-in-one dry reagent immunoassays with fluorescent europium chelate label and time-resolved fluorometry. Clin Chem 42:1196–201

16. Ashraf S, Bhattacharya K, Tian Y, Watterson K (1999) Cytokine and S100B levels in paediatric patients undergoing corrective cardiac surgery with or without total circulatory arrest. Eur J Cardiothorac Surg 16:32–7
17. Donato R (2001) S100: a multigenic family of calcium-modulated proteins of the EF-hand type with intracellular and extracellular functional roles. Int J Biochem Cell Biol 33:637-68
18. Ettinger A, Laumark AB, Ostroff RM, Brundell J, Baumgartner WA, Razumovsky AY (1999) A new optical immunoassay for detection of S-100B protein in whole blood. Ann Thorac Surg 68:2196–201
19. Takahashi M, Chamczuk A, Hong Y, Jackowski G (1999) Rapid and sensitive immunoassay for the measurement of serum S100B using isoform-specific monoclonal antibody. Clin Chem 45:1307–11
20. Missler U, Wiesmann M, Friedrich C, Kaps M (1997) S-100 protein and neuron-specific enolase concentrations in blood as indicators of infarction volume and prognosis in acute ischemic stroke. Stroke 28:1956–60
21. van Engelen BG, Lamers KJ, Gabreels FJ, Wevers RA, van Geel WJ ,Borm GF (1992) Age-related changes of neuron-specific enolase, S-100 protein, and myelin basic protein concentrations in cerebrospinal fluid. Clin Chem 38:813–6
22. Wiesmann M, Missler U, Gottmann D, Gehring S (1998) Plasma S-100b Protein Concentration in Healthy Adults Is Age- and Sex-Independent. Clin Chem 44:1056–1058
23. Anderson RE, Hansson LO, Nilsson O, Dijlai-Merzoug R, Settergren G (2001) High serum S100B levels for trauma patients without head injuries. Neurosurgery 48:1255–8
24. Nilsson O, Andersson I, Nilsson K (1999) Expression of S100ab and S100bb in malignant melanoma. Tumor Biol 20(S2):84

Plasma DNA As A Noninvasive Monitoring Tool For Trauma Patients

Y. M. D. Lo,[1] T. H. Rainer[2]

[1]Departments of Chemical Pathology and [2]Accident & Emergency Medicine Academic Unit, The Chinese University of Hong Kong, Prince of Wales Hospital, Shatin, New Territories, HONG KONG.

Abstract

Introduction

Post-traumatic organ failure is common following severe injury and is an important cause of mortality (1). There is much recent interest in the use of circulating cell-free DNA in the plasma for clinical diagnosis (2). We hypothesize that DNA may be liberated from body tissues into the plasma following trauma and that plasma DNA may be a potentially useful monitoring tool for trauma patients.

Methods

Eighty four patients with acute blunt traumatic injury, requiring admission to the Emergency Resuscitation Room at the Prince of Wales Hospital, and 27 healthy controls were recruited. The total extent of the injury was calculated using an objective Injury Severity Score (ISS) either at the time of discharge, death or at 28 days if the patient was still hospitalized (1). Three mL of peripheral venous blood was collected from each patient at a median time of 60 minutes post-injury.

Plasma DNA was measured using a real-time quantitative polymerase chain reaction assay towards the human *beta-globin* gene as described (3). Plasma DNA concentration was expressed in kilogenome-equivalents/L. One kilogenome-equivalent was defined as the amount of a particular target sequence contained in 1000 diploid human cells.

Results

The median plasma DNA concentrations in the control, minor/moderate trauma ($ISS < 16$; $n = 47$) and major trauma ($ISS \geq 16$; $n = 37$) groups were 3154 kilogenome-equivalents/L, 13818 kilogenome-equivalents/L and 181303 kilogenome-equivalents/L, respectively. The differences between these groups were highly significant (Kruskal-Wallis test, p<0.001). Pairwise comparisons using the Dunn's method reveal significant difference between each constituent pair within these 3 groups (p<0.05).

Plasma DNA concentrations in patients stratified according to acute lung injury (ALI), acute respiratory distress syndrome (ARDS) and death (n=9) are shown in the following table. Patients with adverse outcomes had significantly higher plasma DNA concentrations (11.6 to 12 times) than those who did not develop these complications.

Complications	Median Plasma DNA Concentration (kilogenome-equivalents/L)		Mann-Whitney Rank Sum Test
	With Complication	Without Complication	
ALI (n=6)	398225	33176	p=0.002
ARDS (n=5)	403999	34682	p=0.005
Death (n=9)	315122	26244	p=0.002

Conclusions

This study shows that circulating plasma DNA in the peripheral blood of trauma patients increases early after injury and these increases are related to the development of post-traumatic complications. We believe that plasma DNA may be a valuable tool for the monitoring and prognostication of trauma patients.

References

1. Sauaia A, Moore FA, Moore EE et al. Multiple organ failure can be predicted as early as 12 hours after injury. J Trauma 1998; 45: 291–301.
2. Lo YMD. Circulating nucleic acids in plasma and serum: an overview. Ann NY Acad Sci 2001; 345: 1–7.
3. Lo YMD, Rainer TH, Chan LYS et al. Plasma DNA as a prognostic marker in trauma patients. Clin Chem 2000; 46: 319–23.

Abbreviations

ALI, acute lung injury; ARDS, acute respiratory distress syndrome; OF, organ failure; AIS, Abbreviated Injury Score; ISS, Injury Severity Score; CK, creatine kinase; AST, aspartate aminotransaminase; LDH, lactate dehydrogenase; ROC, Receiver operating characteristic curve

Introduction

Post-traumatic organ failure is common following severe injury and is an important cause of mortality (1). The current hypothesis is that a systemic inflammatory response syndrome follows severe trauma and that the processes eventually lead to organ failure, including acute lung injury (ALI) and the acute respiratory distress syndrome (ARDS) (1). Recently, models have been proposed for the prediction of multiple organ failure as early as 12 hours after injury (1). It would be useful to develop new assays which may allow risk stratification to be made even earlier.

There is much recent interest in the use of circulating cell-free DNA in the plasma for clinical diagnosis (2–4). For example, in patients with cancer, tumor-derived genetic alterations have been found in the plasma and serum (2,3). The analogous phenomenon has also been found during pregnancy, when the unborn fetus has been shown to release its DNA into the plasma and serum of the pregnant mother (4). As an further example of this phenomonen, DNA originating from the donor has been shown to be present in the plasma of recipients of liver and kidney transplantation (5). The clinical applications of these various manifestations of circulating nucleic acids for the purpose of cancer detection, prenatal diagnosis and graft rejection monitoring are being actively pursued in many laboratories in the world.

As DNA is normally expected to reside in the nucleus (with the exception of mitochondrial DNA) and to be essential for cellular functions, it is quite counter-intuitive to find DNA in the plasma. Thus, it has been proposed that DNA is released into the circulation following cell death (6). Along this line of reasoning, we hypothesize that plasma DNA may be clinically useful as a monitoring and prognosticating tool for injurious processes which result in tissue damage and cell death. In this investigation, we attempt to prove this hypothesis by studying if increased amounts of DNA may be released into the plasma following trauma. We further study if plasma DNA may be a potentially useful prognosticating tool for trauma victims.

Materials and Methods

Patients

Eighty four patients who had sustained an acute blunt traumatic injury, were recruited from the Emergency Resuscitation Room at the Prince of Wales Hospital, Hong Kong. These subjects were recruited between April 1996 and September 1999, with informed consent either from the patient or a relative. The project was approved by the Research Ethics Committee of the Chinese University of Hong Kong. Patients aged less than 12 years, pregnant, or subject to drowning, thermal injury, hypothermia and acute drug overdose were excluded. Two out of the 84 patients had a systolic blood pressure of less than 90 mmHg on admission.

The Abbreviated Injury Score (AIS) for individual bodily regions was determined as described (7). The Maximal Abbreviated Injury Score (MAIS) was also determined as described (7). The total extent of the injury was calculated using an objective Injury Severity Score (ISS) either at the time of discharge, death or at 28 days if the patient was still hospitalised (8). The definition of ALI and ARDS was as previously described (9). For classification and regression tree (CART) analysis (see below), we used a catch-all definition under the term 'organ failure' (OF), which included all cases of multiple organ dysfunction syndrome, patients who die, and those with single or multiple organ failure, both within and after 48 hours of injury. Thus, OF includes any patient who developed one or more failed organ systems, as defined by Goris' score (10), at any time between admission and 28 days after injury. Shock index was derived from the first measured pulse and blood pressure readings on arrival in the emergency room (11).

Three mL of peripheral venous blood was collected from each patient into heparinized tubes after they were admitted to the resuscitation room. The median time between injury and blood sampling was 60 minutes (interquartile range: 50 to 100 minutes). At the time of blood sampling, 39 patients had between 500 mL and 1000 mL of intravenous crystalloids; the rest had less than 500 mL. None of the patients had colloids administered prior to the time of blood sampling. The hematocrit was measured on admission as part of the diagnostic workup for each patient. Plasma creatine kinase (CK), aspartate aminotransaminase (AST) and lactate dehydrogenase (LDH) levels were determined using a Dade Behring Dimension® clinical chemistry system. The ISS values, AIS values, MAIS values, outcomes and other clinical parameters were 'blinded' to the laboratory staff carrying out the subsequent plasma DNA analysis. Control blood samples were also obtained from 27 healthy volunteers.

Processing Of Blood Samples

Blood samples were centrifuged at 3000 *g*, and plasma samples were carefully removed from blood collection tubes and transferred into plain polypropylene tubes. Great care was taken to ensure that the cell pellet was undisturbed when plasma samples were removed. The samples were stored at −80 °C or −20 °C until further processing.

DNA Extraction From Plasma Samples

DNA from plasma samples was extracted using a QIAamp Blood Kit (Qiagen, Hilden, Germany) using the "blood and body fluid protocol" as recommended by the manufacturer (2). Four hundred to 800 μL of plasma sample was used for DNA extraction per column. The exact amount used was documented to enable the calculation of target DNA concentration (12).

Real Time Quantitative Polymerase Chain Reaction (PCR)

Theoretical and practical aspects of real time quantitative PCR have been described in detail elsewhere (12–14). Real time quantitative PCR analysis was performed using a PE Applied Biosystems 7700 Sequence Detector (Foster City, CA, U.S.A.). The amplification and product reporting system used was based on the 5' nuclease assay (15) (the TaqMan assay as marketed by Perkin-Elmer) in which the liberation of a fluorescent reporter is coupled to the amplification reaction. A typical run (including blood centrifugation and DNA extraction, followed by real time PCR) took approximately 3 hours.

Plasma DNA was measured using a real time quantitative PCR assay for the *β-globin* gene which is present in all nucleated cells of the body (12). The *β-globin* TaqMan system consisted of the amplification primers beta-globin-354F, 5'-GTG CAC CTG ACT CCT GAG GAG A-3'; beta-globin-455R, 5'-CCT TGA TAC CAA CCT GCC CAG-3'; and a dual labeled fluorescent TaqMan probe beta-globin-402T, 5'-(FAM)AAG GTG AAC GTG GAT GAA GTT GGT GG(TAMRA)-3' (12). The TaqMan probe contained a 3'-blocking phosphate group to prevent probe extension during PCR.

When applied to serial dilutions of human genomic DNA, this real time *β-globin* quantitative PCR assay was able to detect the DNA equivalent from a single cell. The imprecision of this system has been previously reported, with a coefficient of variation of the threshold cycle of 1.1% (12).

The expression of quantitative results was as previously described (12). The unit of kilogenome-equivalents/L was preferred to kilogenome-equivalents/L in accordance with S.I. unit convention. One genome-equivalent was defined as the amount of a particular target sequence contained in a single diploid human cell.

Statistical Analysis

Descriptive statistics and non-parametric data comparison tests were carried out using the SigmaStat 2.0 software. Receiver operating characteristic (ROC) curve analysis was carried out using the MedCalc 5.0 software.

Multivariate analysis was performed using the Classification and Regression Tree (CART) program AnswerTree™ version 2.0 (SPSS). This program used a non-parametric, binary, recursive-partitioning algorithm that yields a tree-structured rule for prediction (16).

The ten variables selected for entry into CART analysis included plasma DNA, plasma albumin, plasma enzymes (CK, AST, LDH), hematocrit, white cell count, injury severity score, maximal abbreviated injury score and shock index.

Results

Plasma DNA Levels And Trauma Severity

The median plasma DNA concentrations in the control, minor/moderate trauma (ISS < 16; n=47) and major trauma (ISS ≥ 16; n=37) groups were 3154 kilogenome-equivalents/L, 13818 kilogenome-equivalents/L and 181303 kilogenome-equivalents/L, respectively (Figure. 1). The differences between these groups were highly significant (Kruskal-Wallis test, $p<0.001$). Pairwise comparisons using the Dunn's method reveal significant difference between each constituent pair within these 3 groups ($p<0.05$). The direct comparison of the individual ISS value with the concentration of plasma DNA revealed a positive correlation, both including (Spearman rank order correlation, $p<0.0005$, $r=0.756$) or excluding (Spearman rank order correlation, $p<0.0005$, $r=0.617$) the control group (ISS = 0). Significant correlations were observed between plasma DNA levels and the AIS values for the head and neck region (Spearman rank order correlation, $p<0.0001$, $r=0.440$), the thorax (Spearman rank order correlation, $p<0.001$, $r=0.520$) and the abdomen (Spearman rank order correlation, $p=0.0002$, $r=0.418$). No significant correlation was observed between plasma DNA levels and the AIS values for the extremities (Spearman rank order correlation, $p=0.136$, $r=0.165$).

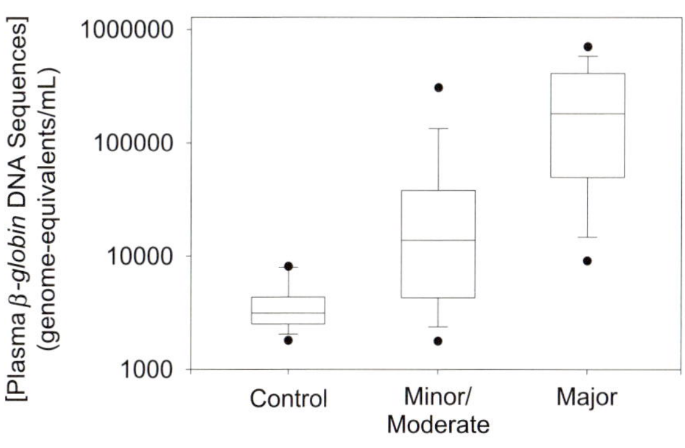

Figure 1. Plasma DNA concentrations in control subjects and trauma patients. The subject categories are shown on the x-axis. Plasma DNA concentrations (kilogenome-equivalents/L) as determined by real time quantitative PCR for the *β-globin* gene are plotted on the y-axis (common logarithmic scale). The lines inside the boxes denote the medians. The boxes mark the interval between the 25th and 75th percentiles. The whiskers denote the interval between the 10th and 90th percentiles. The dots mark the 5th and 95th percentiles.

No significant correlation was observed between the levels of plasma DNA and the admission hematocrit (Spearman rank order correlation, $p=0.311$, $r=-0.111$). The stratification of the patients into those who had received less than 500 mL of intravenous crystalloids and those who had received between 500 mL and 1000 mL by the time of blood sampling revealed no significant difference (Mann-Whitney rank sum test, p=0.25).

With regard to other biochemical markers of tissue injury, positive correlations were observed between plasma DNA and plasma CK (Spearman rank order correlation, p<0.0005, r=0.492), AST (Spearman rank order correlation, p<0.0001, r=0.694) and LDH (Spearman rank order correlation, p<0.0005, r=0.584).

Plasma DNA And Clinical Outcome

To determine if plasma DNA analysis may be used as a prognostic indicator, plasma DNA concentrations amongst groups with different outcomes were compared. Outcomes which were studied include the development of ALI (n=6), ARDS (n=5) and death (n=9). Plasma DNA concentrations in patients stratified according to each of these outcomes are shown in Table 1 which indicates that patients with adverse outcomes had significantly higher plasma DNA concentrations (11.6 to 12 times) than those who did not develop these complications.

Table 1. Plasma DNA concentrations in trauma patients stratified according to outcome, including acute lung injury (ALI), acute respiratory distress syndrome (ARDS) and death.

Complications	Median Plasma DNA Concentration (kilogenome-equivalents/L)		Mann-Whitney Rank Sum Test
	With Complication	Without Complication	
ALI	398225	33176	p=0.002
ARDS	403999	34682	p=0.005
Death	315122	26244	p=0.002

Receiver Operating Characteristic (ROC) Curve Analysis

ROC curve analysis for the use of plasma DNA measurement for predicting ALI, ARDS and death is shown in Figure 2. The areas under the ROC curves for ALI, ARDS and death are, respectively, 0.882 (standard error = 0.091, 95% confidence interval (CI) 0.794–0.942), 0.877 (standard error = 0.102, 95% CI 0.788–0.939) and 0.822 (standard error = 0.088, 95% CI 0.724–0.896).

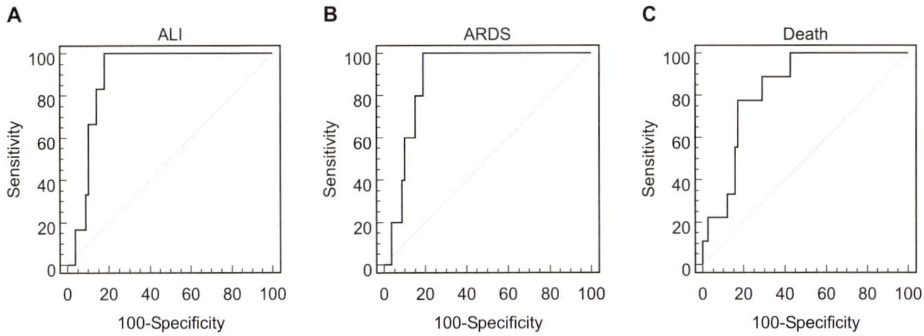

Figure 2. Receiver operating characteristic (ROC) curve analysis of plasma DNA analysis for the prediction of *(A)* acute lung injury (ALI), *(B)* acute respiratory distress syndrome (ARDS) and *(C)* death. The values indicated on the x- and y-axes are expressed in percentages.

For each of these adverse outcomes, plasma DNA of 232719 kilogenome-equivalents/L corresponded to the highest value for the sum of sensitivities and specificities. Using this cut-off, the sensitivities of plasma DNA analysis for the prediction of ALI, ARDS and death were 100% (95% CI, 100–100%), 100% (100–100%) and 78% (40–97%), respectively. The respective specificity figures are 81% (95% CI, 71–89%), 80% (70–88%) and 82% (71–90%).

Classification And Regression Tree (CART) Analysis

To further improve the specificity of plasma DNA-based prediction of clinical outcome, CART analysis was carried out using plasma DNA concentrations and other clinical/laboratory parameters. Clinical information and the complete set of laboratory data were available in 83 of the 84 studied subjects. These 83 individuals were entered for CART analysis. When plasma DNA, AST, ISS and MAIS were entered into the CART program, an optimal model for OF was derived (Table 2). An illustrated example of the recursive partitioning model for predicting OF is shown in Figure 3. The CART-derived algorithm depicted in Table 2 yielded an overall correct classification of 93%. Other combinations were possible but were more complicated and added little to the accuracy of prediction.

Table 2. Classification and Regression Tree (CART) prediction model for posttraumatic organ failure (OF).

	Correct classification rate	
For those who develop OF		
DNA > 140 000 *and* AST > 50†	17/20 (85%)	–
For those who do not develop OF		
DNA ≤ 140 000	55/57 (96.5%)	–
DNA > 140 000 *and* AST ≥ 50†	5/6 (83.3%)	–
Overall correct classification rate	–	**77/83 (92.8%)**
Sensitivity	–	**17/20 (85%)**
Specificity	–	**60/63 (95%)**
Positive predictive value	–	**17/20 (85%)**
Negative predictive value	–	**60/63 (95%)**

† DNA in kilogenome-equivalents/mL; AST, aspartate aminotransaminase in U/L.

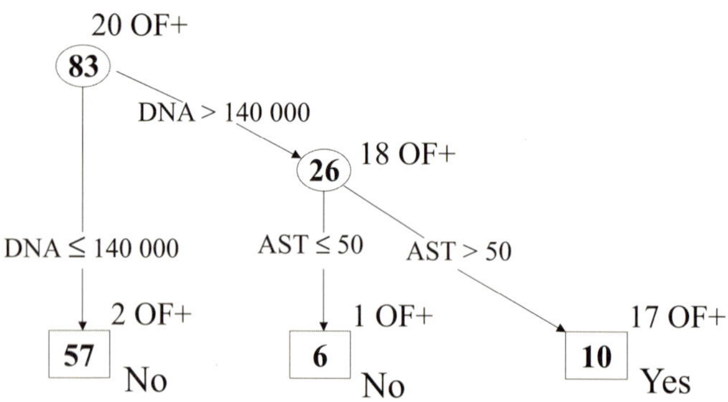

Figure 3. Example of a Classification and Regression Tree for predicting organ failure (OF). AST, aspartate aminotransaminase concentrations in U/L; DNA, plasma DNA concentrations in kilogenome-equivalents/mL

Discussion

This study shows that circulating plasma DNA in the peripheral blood of trauma patients increases early after injury and that these increases are related to the development of post-traumatic complications.We have designed the study such that analysis was performed on a single sample obtained at a median time of 1 hour following trauma, when the physiologic status of the patients was relatively uncomplicated by multiple therapeutic maneuvers, apart from a modest amount (up to 1 L) of intravenous crystalloids.

The mechanisms by circulating DNA is increased following trauma are unclear at present. Theoretically, such an increase may be the result of increased liberation following cell death, or decreased efficiency of DNA clearance mechanisms following injury. In the former case, the cell types (e.g. myocytes and endothelial cells) primarily responsible for DNA liberation remains to be elucidated. It is likely that cell death as a direct result of trauma, or secondarily due to hemodynamic compromise as a result of blood loss, may result in DNA liberation into the circulation. This possibility is supported by the positive correlation between plasma DNA levels and other biochemical markers for tissue injury, namely, CK, AST and LDH. The clearance mechanisms for circulating DNA are poorly understood at present but it is possible that direct damage or hemodynamic compromise of the organ systems normally responsible for circulating DNA clearance may also result in increased levels of plasma DNA.

The comparison between plasma DNA concentrations and the AIS values obtained for the head and neck, thoracic and abdominal regions revealed a positive and significant correlation between these parameters. However, there was no significant correlation between plasma DNA concentrations and the AIS values for the extremities. One interpretation of these results is that the extremities are not the predominant organ systems responsible for the elevation of circulating DNA in trauma patients. On the other hand, the positive correlation between plasma DNA levels and the AIS values for the head and neck, thoracic and abdominal regions support the hypothesis that organ systems in these anatomic regions are responsible for the increased plasma DNA following trauma. Candidate organ systems include the liver, spleen and kidneys which may have a role both in liberating and clearing circulating DNA. For example, evidence of these organs' role in circulating DNA clearance has already been demonstrated in animal experiments (17,18).

As the current study was focussed on blunt trauma, it would be interesting to investigate whether other types of tissue insults, e.g., ischemic, infective, toxic, thermal or radiation injuries may be associated with cell-free DNA liberation into the circulation. These future studies may open up the possibilities that plasma DNA may be used as a general marker for monitoring diverse types of tissue damage. Further work would be required to elucidate the physicochemical characteristics of trauma-associated circulating DNA and to determine whether this type of plasma DNA differs in any fundamental aspects from other circulating DNA species, e.g., fetal DNA (4) and tumor-derived DNA (2,3).

The prediction model obtained following CART analysis offers the possibility that OF may be diagnosed and predicted within 4 to 6 hours of the initial injurious event. The sensitivity and specificity in our study offer an improvement over previous prediction models (1), and the prediction values suggest that this would be an useful rule for early post-traumatic risk stratification. The ability for rapid risk stratification may allow clinicians to make a more rational decision in regard to the type of therapy that is most appropriate for a particular patient.

Recent data indicate that human plasma DNA possesses a short half-life in the circulation (19). The rapid kinetics of plasma DNA suggest that circulating DNA analysis may be useful in monitoring the clinical progress of trauma patients. It is possible that evaluation of the patterns of plasma DNA variation may further enhance the diagnostic accuracy of this type of analysis for predicting adverse clinical outcomes in these patients. There is thus a necessity for future studies to focus on obtaining sequential data from trauma patients. Plasma DNA analysis may also be useful in studying the patients' response to treatment, especially in trials aimed at testing new therapeutic modalities for these patients.

Our current protocol allows the provision of plasma DNA results within 3 hours of blood sampling. This rapidity is achieved by the use of a simple column-based DNA extraction method and the utilization of real time PCR analysis which does not require any post-amplification manipulation. With the recent development of rapid capillary-based instrumentation for quantitative PCR analysis (20), this time could be further reduced to 90 minutes, thus further enhancing the potential clinical usefulness of this assay in accident and emergency departments.

Acknowledgments

YMDL is supported by the Hong Kong Research Grants Council, the Industrial Support Fund and the Direct Grants Scheme from The Chinese University of Hong Kong. We thank LYS Chan, N Lam, RA Cocks, NM Hjelm, CW Lam, LCW Lit and SMH Yu for help during the course of this project.

References

1. Sauaia A, Moore FA, Moore EE, Norris JM, Lezotte DC, Hamman RF (1998). Multiple organ failure can be predicted as early as 12 hours after injury. J Trauma;45:291–301.
2. Chen XQ, Stroun M, Magnenat JL, et al (1996). Microsatellite alterations in plasma DNA of small cell lung cancer patients. Nat Med;2:1033–5.
3. Nawroz H, Koch W, Anker P, Stroun M, Sidransky D (1996). Microsatellite alterations in serum DNA of head and neck cancer patients. Nat Med;2:1035–7.
4. Lo YMD, Corbetta N, Chamberlain PF, et al (1997). Presence of fetal DNA in maternal plasma and serum. Lancet;350:485–7.
5. Lo YMD, Tein MSC, Pang CCP, Yeung CK, Tong KL, Hjelm NM (1998). Presence of donor-specific DNA in plasma of kidney and liver-transplant recipients. Lancet;351:1329–30.

6. Fournie GJ, Courtin JP, Laval F, et al. (1995). Plasma DNA as a marker of cancerous cell death. Investigations in patients suffering from lung cancer and in nude mice bearing human tumours. Cancer Lett;91:221–7.
7. Committee on Medical Aspects of Automotive Safety (1971). Rating the severity of tissue damage. I. The abbreviated scale. JAMA;215:277–80.
8. Boyd CR, Tolson MA, Copes WS (1987). Evaluating trauma care: the TRISS method. Trauma Score and the Injury Severity Score. J Trauma;27:370–8.
9. Bernard GR, Artigas A, Brigham KL, et al. (1994). Report of the American-European consensus conference on ARDS: definitions, mechanisms, relevant outcomes and clinical trial coordination. The Consensus Committee. Intensive Care Med;20:225–32.
10. Goris RJ, te Boekhorst TP, Nuytinck JK, Gimbrere JS (1985). Multiple-organ failure. Generalized autodestructive inflammation? Arch Surg;120:1109–15.
11. Rady MY, Rivers EP, Martin GB, Smithline H, Appelton T, Nowak RM (1992). Continuous central venous oximetry and shock index in the emergency department: use in the evaluation of clinical shock. Am J Emerg Med;10:538–41.
12. Lo YMD, Tein MS, Lau TK, et al (1998). Quantitative analysis of fetal DNA in maternal plasma and serum: implications for noninvasive prenatal diagnosis. Am J Hum Genet;62:768–75.
13. Heid CA, Stevens J, Livak KJ, Williams PM (1996). Real time quantitative PCR. Genome Res;6:986–94.
14. Luthra R, McBride JA, Cabanillas F, Sarris A (1998). Novel 5' exonuclease-based real-time PCR assay for the detection of t(14;18)(q32;q21) in patients with follicular lymphoma. Am J Pathol;153:63–8.
15. Holland PM, Abramson RD, Watson R, Gelfand DH (1991). Detection of specific polymerase chain reaction product by utilizing the 5'——3' exonuclease activity of Thermus aquaticus DNA polymerase. Proc Natl Acad Sci U S A;88:7276–80.
16. Brieman I, Friedman JH, Olshen RA, Stone CJ (1993). Classification and Regression Trees. New York: Chapman and Hall.
17. Tsumita T, Iwanaga M (1963). Fate of injected deoxyribonucleic acid in mice. Nature;198:1088–9.
18. Chused TM, Steinberg AD, Talal N (1972). The clearance and localization of nucleic acids by New Zealand and normal mice. Clin Exp Immunol;12:465–76.
19. Lo YMD, Zhang J, Leung TN, Lau TK, Chang AM, Hjelm NM (1999). Rapid clearance of fetal DNA from maternal plasma. Am J Hum Genet;64:218–24.
20. Wittwer CT, Ririe KM, Andrew RV, David DA, Gundry RA, Balis UJ (1997). The LightCycler: a microvolume multisample fluorimeter with rapid temperature control. BioTechniques; 22:176–81.

Clinical Application Of A Highly Sensitive Immuno-Polymerase Chain Reaction For Serum Tumor Necrosis Factor α

D Kobayashi, K Saito, M Komatsu, N Watanabe

Sapporo Medical University, Sapporo, JAPAN.

Abstract

Introduction

Tumor necrosis factor α (TNF-α) plays an important role in inflammation by eliminating foreign substances, e. g., bacteria and grafts, through the activation of chemotaxis and phagocytosis, induction and release of oxygen free radicals and degranulation of monocyte/macrophages. However, it is unclear whether measurement of serum TNF-α can be useful in understanding various pathophysiologic processes, since low concentrations of TNF-α including those in healthy donors could not be measured by the methods used in previous studies. In this study, therefore, we determined reference values in normal healthy donors and measured serum TNF-α levels in diseases such as inflammatory bowel diseases (IBD) and Duchennne muscular dystrophy (DMD), using a highly sensitive immuno-polymerase chain reaction established in our laboratory (1–3).

Methods

Serum samples in this study were collected from age-matched 54 healthy blood donors, 54 samples from 36 patients with IBD, and 65 samples from DMD patients. The healthy blood donors were selected randomly from workers in our hospital who had been determined to be healthy by clinical examination. Immuno-PCR and ELISA was performed according to our method described previously (1). The detection limit of this immuno-PCR has been approximately $5x10^4$-fold lower than that of the ELISA for TNF-α, as described in our previous report (1).

Results

The serum concentration in IBD patients overall (mean, 56.660 ng/L) was approximately 2000 times that in healthy donors (mean, 0.027 ng/L), (mean excess for ulcerative colitis, 1100 times; for Crohn's Disease, 7700 times). Of the 54 samples, 50 (93%) had TNF-α concentrations below the detection limit of conventional ELISA.

In addition, serum TNFα was higher in the active stage of IBD than in the inactive stage. In UC patients, mean CRP concentrations remained below the detection limit in 37 of 46 samples (80%).

The mean TNFα concentration in DMD patients (27.8 ng/L) was approximately 1000 times higher than that in healthy donors. The mean TNFα concentration in patients under 20 years old who showed high creatine kinase (CK) and myoglobin (Mb) concentrations was approximately 5 times higher than in the patients over 20 years old, showing that elevation of serum TNFα is particularly marked in the early progressive stage of the disease.

Conclusions

These studies demonstrated that sensitive measurement of serum TNFα could provide or important pathophysiologic marker for presence and activity of IBD and DMD.

References

1. Saito K, Kobayashi D, Sasaki M, et al. Detection of human serum tumor necrosis factor-a in healthy donors, using a highly sensitive immuno-PCR assay. Clin Chem 1999;45: 665–9.
2. Saito K, Kobayashi D, Komatsu M et al. A sensitive assay of tumor necrosis factor alpha in sera from Duchenne muscular dystrophy patients. Clin Chem 2000;46: 1703–4.
3. Komatsu M, Kobayashi D, Saito K et al. Tumor necrosis factor in serum of inflammatory bowel disease as measured by a highly sensitive immuno polymerase chain reaction. Clin Chem 2001;47: 1297–301.

Introduction

Tumor necrosis factor α (TNFα) is a multifunctional cytokine initially identified as a monocyte/macrophage-derived serum protein mediating necrosis of solid tumors in mice (1, 2). TNFα has various physiologic activities that not only affect tumor cells, but normal cells as well (3, 4). Tumor necrosis factor α (TNFα) plays an important role in inflammation and degenerative process by eliminating foreign substances, e. g., bacteria and grafts, through the activation of chemotaxis and phagocytosis, induction and release of oxygen free radicals and degranulation of monocyte/macrophages. Several inflammatory, autoimmune, and neuromuscular diseases are thought to be due to excessive TNFα activity. However, it is unclear whether measurement of serum TNFα can be useful in understanding various pathophysiologic processes, since low concentrations of TNFα including those in healthy donors could not be measured by the methods used in previous studies. We recently established a highly sensitive method for measurement of TNFα in serum by an immuno-polymerase chain reaction (PCR) assay (5), which has a sensitivity $5x10^4$ times greater than that of a conventional enzyme-linked immunosorbent assay (ELISA). In this study, therefore, we determined reference values in normal healthy donors and measured serum TNF-α levels in diseases such as inflammatory bowel diseases (IBD) and Duchenne muscular dystrophy (DMD), using a highly sensitive immuno-polymerase chain reaction (5–7).

Methods

Serum samples

Samples in this study were collected from 29 patients with Ulcerative colitis (mean age, 39 years; range 20–73 years), 7 patients with Crohn's disease (mean age, 39 years; range 23–68 years), and 65 patients with DMD (mean age, 20.7 years; range 7–46 years). Fifty-four healthy blood donors (mean age, 39 years; range 25–61 years) were selected randomly from workers in our hospital who had been determined to be healthy by clinical examination. Serum samples were stored at –80°C until being assayed.

Human recombinant TNFa and antibodies

Human recombinant TNF, mouse anti-human recombinant TNF-α monoclonal antibody (mAb), and rabbit anti-human recombinant TNF-α polyclonal antibody (pAb) for ELISA and immuno-PCR assay were generously provided by ASAHI Chemical Industry Co., Tokyo, Japan.

Enzyme-linked immunosorbent assay (ELISA)

ELISA was performed according to our method described previously (5). The absorbance of the sample was determined at 492 nm in an ELISA reader EAR400 (SLT - Labinstruments, Gesellschaft M, B, H, Salzburg, Austria). The detection limit of this ELISA was 50 ng/L, as determined by triplicate measurements and represented by the absorbance at 492 nm.

Immuno-Polymerase Chain Reaction (Immuno-PCR)

Immuno-PCR was performed according to our method described previously (5). The limit of detection this immuno-PCR has been approximately $5x10^4$ times -fold lower than that of the ELISA for TNF-α, as described in our previous report (5). The detection limit of this immuno-PCR has been approximately $5x10^4$ -fold lower than that of the ELISA for TNF-α, as described in our previous report (5).

Results

Serum TNF-α concentrations in healthy donors and IBD patients

Of the 54 patients, 50 (93%) had TNF-α concentrations below the detection limit of conventional ELISA; their serum TNF-α concentration was measured by immuno-PCR. The serum concentration in IBD patients overall (mean, 56.660 ng/L) was approximately 2000 times that in healthy donors (mean, 0.027 ng/L) (Figure 1). Mean concentrations in Ulcerative colitis (UC) and Crohn's disease (CD) patients were 1100 and 7700 times higher than in healthy donors, respectively. In addition, the mean concentration in active UC (48.570 ng/L) was 7.5 times that in inactive UC (6.495), while the mean concentration in active CD (404.760 ng/L) was and 34 times higher than in inactive cases (11.967 ng/L).

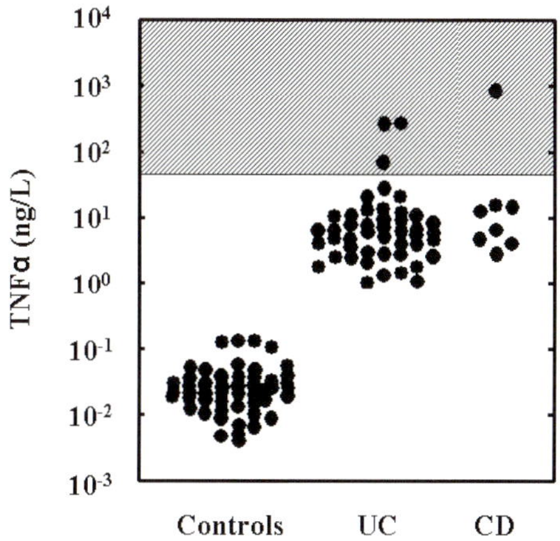

Figure 1. Comparison of serum tumor necrosis factor (TNF) α concentrations between 54 healthy blood donors and 36 patients with inflammatory bowel disease (54 samples; 46 for ulcerative colitis, 8 for Crohn's disease). Shaded area indicates the range of detectability by enzyme-linked immunosorbent assay (ELISA).

TNF-α concentrations in serial samples including active and inactive stages of UC

In six UC patients, serum samples could be obtained during both inactive and active stages. In five of six patients, serum TNF-α concentration in the active stage was notably higher than in the inactive stage (Figure 2). However, TNF-α concentrations in four of these five active-stage samples remained below the detection limit of ELISA.

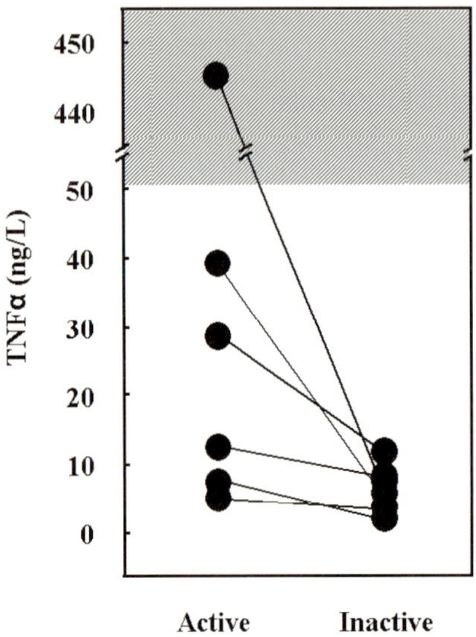

Figure 2. Comparison of serum tumor necrosis factor (TNF) α concentrations between active and inactive stages in six patients with ulcerative colitis. Shaded area indicates the range of detectability by enzyme-linked immunosorbent assay (ELISA).

Correlation between TNFα and C-reactive protein in IBD patients

All of the IBD patients showed an elevated TNF-α concentration, while mean CRP concentrations remained below the detection limit in some cases (Table 1).

Table 1. Tumor necrosis factor (TNF-α) and C-reactive protein (CRP) in patients with inflammatory bowel disease.

Ulcerative Colitis (n=46)				Chron's Disease (n=8)			
		TNF-α (ng/L)[a]				TNF-α (ng/L)	
		< 0.81	≥ 0.81			< 0.81	≥ 0.81
CPR[b] (mg/dl)	< 0.30	0 (0%)	37 (80%)	CPR (mg/dl)	< 0.30	0 (0%)	2 (25%)
	≥ 0.30	0 (0%)	9 (20%)		≥ 0.30	0 (0%)	6 (75%)

[a] 0.081 ng/l represents the mean+2SD of TNF-α measurements in control subjects.
[b] The corresponding value for CRP is 0.3 mg/dL.

This was especially notable in UC patients, whose CRP concentrations were below the detection limit in 37 of 46 cases (80%).

Serum TNFα concentrations in DMD patients and healthy subjects

The mean value in DMD patients (27.8 ng/L) was approximately 1000 times higher than that in healthy subjects (0.027 ng/L) (Figure 3). Fifty-seven of the DMD patients (87.7%) had a TNFα concentration below the detection limit of a conventional ELISA.

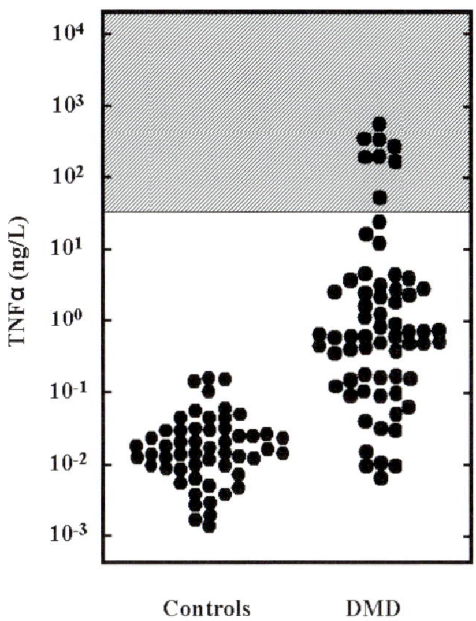

Figure 3. Comparison of tumor necrosis factor α (TNFα) concentrations between sera from 54 healthy subjects and 65 Duchenne muscular dystrophy (DMD) patients by immuno-polymerase chain reaction (PCR). The shaded area shows the range in which TNFα could also be detected by enzyme-linked immunosorbent assay (ELISA).

Serum concentrations of TNFα and other biochemical parameter of DMD patients in two age groups

Patients younger than 20 years old showed a much higher mean CK concentration (2838.0 IU/L) than patients over 20 years old (351.2 IU/L). Mb concentration in patients under 20 years old (405.6 ng/mL) also was higher than that in the cases over 20 years old (66.1 ng/mL). These results indicate the progression of muscle destruction in young patients with DMD. The mean TNFα concentration in the patients under 20 years old (60.7 ng/L) was approximately 5 times higher than that in patients over 20 years old (12.9 ng/L), showing that elevation of serum TNFα is particularly marked in the early progressive stage of the disease (Table 2). In addition, the mean TNFα concentration in the patients under 20 years old was significantly higher than that in normal healthy subjects ($P < 0.05$ by Student's *t*-test after analysis of variance (ANOVA). However, no significant correlation was detected between TNF-α concentration and biochemical parameters such as CK and Mb in the total of 65 DMD patients, nor was a correlation found in DMD patients under 20 years old (Figure 4).

Table 2. Serum TNF-α concentration in DMD Patients was measured by immuno-PCR

	Total	Under 20 yrs	Over 20 yrs
Total Number	65	29	36
Positive Case[a]	52	24	28
Percent Positive	80.0	82.8	77.8
Mean TNF-α (ng/L)	27.8	60.7	12.9

Serum TNF-α concentrations in DMD patients were measured by immuno-PCR.
[a] Serum samples revealed TNF-α concentration in which the mean±SD Value did not overlap that of controls.

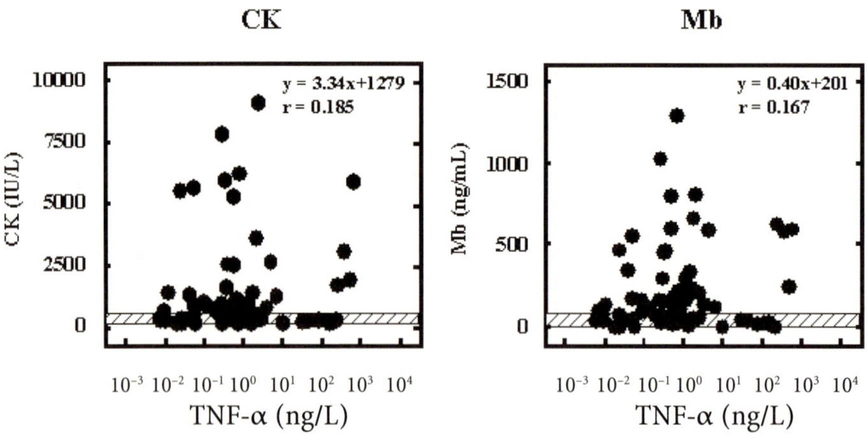

Figure 4. Relationships between serum concentrations of tumor necrosis factor α (TNF-α) and creatine kinase (CK) or myoglobin (Mb) in patients with Duchenne muscular dystrophy (DMD). The shaded area shows the normal range (CK 71 to 220 IU/L; Mb <70 ng/mL).

Conclusions

The pathophysiologic significance of TNF-α in IBD is poorly understood because of difficulties in measuring charges in the serum concentrations ordinarily present in IBD. Using immuno-PCR, we clarified that the mean serum concentration of TNF-α in IBD patients was strikingly higher than in controls. Whether serum TNF-α concentrations differ between UC and CD has not been known. In this study, mean serum TNF-α concentrations in UC and CD were 1100 and 7700 times those in healthy donors, respectively. Some investigators have previously demonstrated that TNF-α-positive cells were more numerous in submucosa and lamina propria from CD patients than in specimens from UC patients, and that TNF-α mRNA expression of mucosal tissues in CD patients was higher than in UC patients (8, 9). A recent study has suggested that Th-1 cytokines induced by TNF-α are important in the pathogenesis of IBD, especially CD (10). The distinctly greater TNF-α elevation found in our CD sera support this view. In the present study, serum TNF-α concentrations in the active stage were approximately 7.5 and 34 times those in inactive stage of UC and CD, respectively. However, the degree to which serum TNF-α concentration decreases in the inactive stage of disease, remained unclear. Fortunately we had sera obtained in both active and inactive stages to measure TNF-α in six individual patients with UC. A difference in serum TNF-α concentration was evident between inactive and active stages in almost all of these serially sampled patients; this difference could not be detected by conventional ELISA. Furthermore, TNF-α concentration in inactive stages of all cases remained higher than that in the healthy subjects. These results suggest that TNF-α could aid diagnosis of disease and assessment of activity in individual patients with IBD. In addition, we compared the frequency with which serum TNF-α and CRP concentrations were increased in UC and CD. Respectively 80 and 25% of UC and CD samples without detectable CRP nonetheless showed elevated TNF-α concentrations. Schreiber et al. recently reported that acute relapse within 1 year could be predicted by increased secretion of TNF-α measured by ELISA, but not by increased CRP concentration (11). Our sensitive assay may further enhance predictive ability and shed light on pathogenesis.

Serum TNF-α measurement in DMD patients have not been informative because of poor detectability by conventional methods. Using a highly sensitive immuno-PCR method, we presently demonstrated a mean concentration of serum TNF-α in DMD patients that was 1000 times higher than that in healthy subjects. Further, we found that elevation of serum TNF-α is particularly marked in the early progressive stage of the disease; the mean TNF-α concentration in patients under 20 years old was approximately 5 times higher than in patients over 20 years old. Previous findings suggested that serum TNF-α concentrations could be elevated as a result of muscle fiber destruction (12, 13). However, we found no significant correlation between the serum concentrations of TNF-α and those of CK or Mb in the present study, arguing against such an explanation. Considering findings from various studies, TNF-α is likely to play an important but presently undetermined pathophysiologic role in DMD. Previous reports have indicated that sudden death from thrombotic disease can occur in DMD patients, in addition to the usual deaths from respiratory and heart failure (14-16). TNF-α is well known to activate the coagulation system. It was speculated that TNF-α elevations in lower concentrations which could not be detected by conventional ELISA may predict not only steady progression but also the progressive and sudden change of disease state such a hypercoagulable state in DMD patients. In addition, in eight of the present cases the serum TNF-α concentration was high enough to be measured by a conventional ELISA. Among these patients, four who were younger than 20 years old showed particularly high TNF-α concentrations, and had progressive difficulty in walking in the weeks following examination. These observations suggested that TNF-α may participate in unusual but acute progression of DMD.

Taken together, it was clarified that sensitive measurement of serum TNF-α could provide or important pathophysiologic marker for presence and activity of inflammatory and neuromuscular diseases such as IBD and DMD.

References

1. Carswell EA, Old LJ, Kassel RL, Green S, Fiore N, Williamson B. An endotoxin-induced serum factor that causes necrosis of tumors. Proc Natl Acad Sci USA 1975;72:3666–70.
2. Helson L, Helson C, Green S. Effect of murine tumor necrosis factor on heterotransplanted human tumors. Exp Cell Biol 1979;47:53–60.
3. Hanemaaijer R, Sorsa T, Konttinen YT, Ding Y, Sutinen M, Visser H, et al. Matrix metalloproteinase-8 is expressed in rheumatoid synovial fibroblasts and endothelial cells. Regulation by tumor necrosis factor-alpha and doxycycline. J Biol Chem 1997;272:31504–9.
4. Ohmori Y, Schreiber RD, Hamilton TA. Synergy between interferon-gamma and tumor necrosis factor-alpha in transcriptional activation is mediated by cooperation between signal transducer and activator of transcription 1 and nuclear factor kappa B. J Biol Chem 1997;272:14899–907.
5. Saito K, Kobayashi D, Sasaki M, et al (1999). Detection of human serum tumor necrosis factor-a in healthy donors, using a highly sensitive immuno-PCR assay. Clin Chem 45: 665–9.
6. Saito K, Kobayashi D, Komatsu M et al (2000). A sensitive assay of tumor necrosis factor alpha in sera from Duchenne muscular dystrophy patients. Clin Chem 46: 1703–4.
7. Komatsu M, Kobayashi D, Saito K et al (2001). Tumor necrosis factor in serum of inflammatory bowel disease as measured by a highly sensitive immuno polymerase chain reaction. Clin Chem 47: 1297–301.
8. Dionne S, Hiscott J, D'agata I, et al. Quantitative PCR analysis of TNF-α and IL-1ß mRNA levels in pediatric IBD mucosal biopsies. Digest Dis Sci 1997; 42: 1557–66.
9. Murch SH, Braegger CP, Walker-Smith JA, et al. Location of tumour necrosis factor a by immunohistochemistry in chronic inflammatory bowel disease. Gut 1993; 34: 1705–9.
10. Plevy SE, Landers CJ, Prehn J, et al. A role for TNF a and mucosal T helper-1 cytokine in the pathogenesis of Crohn's disease. J Immunol 1997; 159: 6276–82.
11. Schreiber S, Nikolaus S, Hampe J, et al. Tumor necrosis factor a and interleukin 1 ß in relapse of Crohn's disease. LANCET 1999; 353: 459–61.
12. Lundberg I, Brengman JM, Engel AG. Analysis of cytokine expression in muscle in inflammatory myopathies, Duchenne dystrophy, and non-weak controls. J Neuroimmunol 1995; 63: 9–16.
13. Tews DS, Goebel HH. Cytokine expression profile in idiopathic inflammatory myopathies. J Neuropath Exp Neur 1996; 55: 342–7.
14. Gaffney JF, Kingston WJ, Metlay LA, Gramiak R. Left ventricular thrombus and systemic emboli complicating the cardiomyopathy of Duchenne's muscular dystrophy. Arch Neurol 1989; 46: 1249–52.
15. Berko BA, Swift M. X-linked dilated cardiomyopathy. New Engl J Med 1987; 316: 1186–91.
16. Chenard AA, Becane HM, Tertrain F, Kermadec JM, Weiss YA. Ventricular arrhythemia in Duchenne muscular dystrophy: prevalence, significance and prognosis. Neuromuscular Disord 1993; 3: 201–6.

Rapid And Reliable Detection Of Fungemia By Polymerase Chain Reaction

U. H. Tirodker, J. P. Nataro, K. D. Fairchild

Department of Pediatrics, University of Maryland School of Medicine, Baltimore, MD, USA

Abstract

Introduction

Fungal infections are a major cause of morbidity and mortality in critically ill patients, especially if treatment is delayed. Blood culture has failed to detect 40–50% of autopsy proven invasive fungal disease and may take 3–5 days to become positive. Polymerase chain reaction (PCR) amplification of highly conserved 18s ribosomal DNA sequences present in multiple fungal species may permit a rapid and sensitive detection of fungemia in neonatal and pediatric ICU patients with suspected sepsis.

Methods

Between 0.2-0.5 mL of whole blood was collected simultaneously with blood culture in pediatric and neonatal ICU patients with suspected sepsis. 0.5 mL of blood was collected from 15 healthy volunteers, as a control group. Samples were pretreated with proteinase K and lyticase, DNA was extracted and the gene for fungal 18 s ribosomal DNA was amplified as described by Einsele at al (1), yielding a 482-503 base pair product, depending on the fungal species. PCR products were analyzed by agarose gel electrophoresis. The sensitivity of the assay was determined using blood spiked with serial dilutions of Candida albicans and purified candida DNA.

Results

Seventy samples were collected from 63 patients (17 PICU, 46 NICU). Nine samples had a positive blood culture for Candida species (6 C.albicans, 1 C.glabrata, 2 mixed C.albicans and C.krusei) and of these all were PCR positive. Of the 4 samples positive for malassezia furfur by culture, only 1 was PCR positive. Of the 57 blood samples with negative fungal culture, 44 were PCR negative. Of the 13 PCR positive/culture negative patients, 6 had concurrent or prior evidence of fungal infection (2 had candiduria, 1 had intestinal perforation with candida peritonitis, 3 were on Amphotericin for previous candidemia). Of the 15 healthy adult controls, 2 were PCR positive (contamination rate of 13%).

Conclusions

PCR for 18s ribosomal DNA was 100% sensitive in the detection of candidemia in neonatal and pediatric ICU patients with suspected sepsis. With further refinement of the method to decrease the false positive rate, this method may enable rapid and reliable detection of fungemia in critically ill children.

Reference

1. Einsele H, Holger H, Roller G et al. Detection and Identification of Fungal Pathogens in Blood by Using Molecular Probes. Journal of Clinical Microbiology, June 1997, p.1353–1360.

Key words: Candida sepsis, polymerase chain reaction, bloodstream infection, neonatal and pediatric intensive care

Introduction

Disseminated *Candida* infection is an increasingly important cause of mortality and morbidity in neonatal and pediatric intensive care unit patients (1). Increased survival of very low birthweight infants and other immunocompromised patients, as well as increasing use of indwelling intravascular catheters, broad spectrum antibiotics, steroids, and parenteral alimentation have contributed to an increase in *Candida* sepsis over the last decade (2–4). A recent survey of very low birth weight (less than 1500 gram) infants revealed that fungal species, predominantly *Candida albicans*, were responsible for 9% of all cases of late onset sepsis with a 28% mortality (5), Another study found a ten-fold increase in the incidence of invasive candidiasis among hospitalized neonates in the last fifteen years (6).

Since *Candida* has a propensity for deep tissue invasion, severe morbidities, including meningoencephalitis, endophthalmitis, osteomyelitis, and endocarditis, are not uncommon. Mortality from disseminated fungal infection is approximately 20 to 30% in NICU and PICU patients (7–9) but may increase to greater than 50% if treatment is delayed (2,10,11). Early detection of fungal sepsis and institution of appropriate therapy has been shown to improve patient outcome (2,11). Fraser et. al. reported that patients with candidemia of more than two days' duration prior to initiation of antifungal therapy had a two-fold higher mortality than those who were treated more promptly (12). Early removal of central venous catheters in neonates and children with candidemia is also associated with significantly decreased mortality and morbidity (2,13,14).

Early and reliable detection of disseminated *Candida* infection is crucial yet problematic. Blood culture detection of candidemia may take three to five days and is often falsely negative. In adults, sensitivity of routine blood culture has been reported to be as low as 50% for detection of autopsy-proven disseminated fungal infection (12) and in neonates, up to thirty percent of all cases of systemic candidiasis are not diagnosed until autopsy (1,15). Because of these impediments to detection of *Candida* sepsis and the high morbidity and mortality associated with delayed treatment, neonatal and pediatric intensive care unit patients are often treated empirically with anti-fungal agents, with attendant risks of toxicity and emergence of drug resistance.

Detection of *Candida* DNA by polymerase chain reaction (PCR) may provide a rapid and reliable screen for candidemia in high-risk patients. PCR amplification of the highly conserved multicopy 18s ribosomal RNA gene present in multiple fungal species but not in bacterial or human DNA, has been developed and tested in the clinical setting (16–18). Einsele et. al. showed that PCR amplification of the 18sRNA gene in the blood of neutropenic cancer patients was highly sensitive when compared with blood culture for detection of candidemia. Furthermore, in many cases the PCR was positive several days before detection of fungemia by blood culture (16,17). We therefore sought to compare 18s ribosomal RNA PCR with blood culture to assess its value in early and reliable detection of fungemia in neonatal and pediatric intensive care unit patients with suspected infection.

Methods

Study Population and Blood Collection

The study was carried out in a 40-bed, level 3 NICU and 18-bed, level 3 PICU from November 1999 through November 2000. Every patient in the NICU and PICU with suspected sepsis was eligible for inclusion. When a patient was undergoing blood culture for suspected infection, excess blood (from 0.2 to 0.5 mL) remaining in the sterile catheter or syringe was collected in an EDTA-containing tube and frozen at -20°C. The Hospital Institutional Review Board determined the study to be exempt from any requirement for consent because of the small volume of waste blood collected. Patients were classified as low, medium or high index of suspicion (IOS) for septicemia based on the judgment of the clinicians involved in the patient's care at the time the blood culture was obtained. Criteria for determining IOS included, but were not limited to, temperature instability, hemodynamic compromise, respiratory deterioration, abnormal white blood cell count or differential, and elevated C-reactive protein. Results of fungal PCR were not made available to the clinicians caring for the patients. Fifteen healthy adults served as a control group from whom 0.5 mL of blood was collected for fungal PCR.

Blood culture

Blood was inoculated for culture into Pediatric Plus bottles (Becton Dickinson Diagnostic Instrument Systems, Sparks, MD) which were monitored on a BACTEC 9240 automated system for 5 days unless a specific request was made to hold the culture as long as fourteen days. Positive fungal blood cultures were examined microscopically, subcultured on blood, chocolate and Sabouraud's agar and then inoculated on a Vitek yeast card for species identification according to standard methods.

Sample DNA extraction

DNA extraction and PCR were performed using a modification of the method described by Einsele (16,18). Patient and healthy control samples (0.2 to 0.5 mL) were treated with red cell lysis buffer (10 mM Tris [pH 7.6], 5 mM $MgCl_{2,}$ 10 mM NaCl) for 10 min at 37°C and centrifuged for 10 min at 5000 × g. White cell lysis buffer (10 mM Tris [pH 7.6], 10 mM EDTA, 50 mM NaCl, 1% SDS, and 150 µg/ml proteinase K) was added and the samples incubated at 65°C for 1 hour. Following centrifugation, fungal cell walls were lysed by suspending the pellet in lysis buffer (50 mm Tris [pH 7.6], 1 mM EDTA, 28 mM β-mercaptoethanol and 3 units of lyticase [Sigma, St. Louis, MO]). After incubation at 37°C for one hour, 10% SDS was added and incubation continued at 65°C for 20 minutes. Protein precipitation with potassium acetate was followed by DNA extraction with isopropanol. DNA was stored at –80°C and assayed in batch by PCR. In order to verify successful DNA extraction from the small blood volumes obtained for the study, an initial PCR was performed on all samples for the constitutively-expressed GAPDH gene. Of eighty samples initially collected, successful DNA extraction was confirmed in seventy and others were excluded from analysis. None of the ten patient samples excluded from the study were positive for fungus by culture.

Candida culture and determination of *in vitro* PCR and blood culture sensitivity

A single colony of *C. albicans* (adult patient isolate) was swirled in 1 mL of thioglycolate broth and agitated at 35°C for 48 hours. The inoculum was centrifuged for 5 min at 12,000 × g and the pellet washed twice with sterile normal saline. The fungal saline suspension was adjusted photometrically to a concentration of 10^7 CFU/mL. The suspension was then serially diluted tenfold (10^6 to 10^0 Colony forming units, CFU/mL) and plated on Sabouraud-dextrose medium for confirmation of colony count. Serial dilutions of *C. albicans* were spiked into 1 ml of whole blood from a healthy volunteer. Half of each spiked blood sample was inoculated into a Pediatric Plus culture bottle (Becton Dickinson) and the other half subjected to sample DNA extraction as described above, followed by PCR amplification.

Candida DNA extraction

The washed pellet of *C. albicans* prepared as described above was resuspended in 500 ml of lysis buffer (50 mM Tris [pH 7.5], 10 mM EDTA, 0.5% β-mercaptoethanol and 0.3 mg/ml Zymolase [ICN, Costa Mesa, California] and incubated at 37°C for one hour. Proteinase K (Boehringer Mannheim, Mannheim, Germany) 50 μg/ml in 1% SDS was added and the mixture incubated for one hour at 56°C, then heated to 95°C for 5 min. DNA was extracted with phenol-chloroform-isoamyl alcohol (25:24:1) and precipitated with isopropanol (19). DNA quantitation was performed by spectrophotometric measurement of absorbance at 260 nm. Serial dilutions of purified *C. albicans* DNA (4.5 nanograms to 0.45 femtograms) in sterile normal saline were prepared and subjected to PCR.

Polymerase chain reaction

Five microlitres of extracted DNA was amplified in a 50-μL reaction mixture with 1 × PCR buffer (10 mM Tris [pH 8.8], 1.5 mM $MgCl_2$, 25 mM KCl and 0.5 units Perfect Match Polymerase Enhancer, [Stratagene, La Jolla, California]), 100 μM of deoxynucleotide triphosphates, and 30 picomoles of each primer (forward primer 5' - ATT GGA GGG CAA GTC TGG TG -3', reverse primer 5' - CCG ATC CCT AGT CGG CAT AG-3'). These primers amplify a 482-503 base pair fragment of the 18s rRNA gene, depending on the fungal species(16). The amplification was performed in a Perkin-Elmer 480 Thermocycler [Perkin-Elmer Corporation, Norwalk, CT]). The amplification consisted of a hot start followed by 35 cycles of 94°C for 30 seconds, 62°C for 1 minute, and 72°C for 2 minutes, followed by a final extension at 72°C for 5 minutes. PCR products were analyzed on an ethidium bromide-stained 2% agarose gel. Gels were analyzed for presence of the fungal PCR product by two independent observers blinded to blood culture results and patient information.

To minimize the risk of contamination, sample preparation and PCR analysis were carried out in separate rooms. Sterile gloves and barrier tips were used for all steps in the protocol. Labware, solutions, and workspaces were autoclaved, UV irradiated, and/or HCl-washed, as appropriate. To monitor for contamination, negative controls (sterile water and whole blood from a healthy volunteer) were used in each extraction and amplification. Purified *C. albicans* DNA served as a positive control.

Results

Patient Characteristics

Over a twelve month period, DNA was extracted from 70 eligible blood samples collected from 63 patients (46 NICU, 17 PICU). Of these samples, 53 were from a peripheral blood draw, 13 from a central venous line, and 4 from an arterial line. Index of suspicion for septicemia was high in 29 (41%) cases, medium in 17 (25%), and low in 24 (34%). Forty-seven samples (67%) were from patients on antibiotics and seven samples (10%) were from patients on antifungal agents at the time of collection.

Sensitivity of 18s rRNA PCR and experimental blood culture for detection of C. albicans

The lower limit of PCR detection of purified *C. albicans* DNA was 45 picograms. corresponding to approximately 100 organisms per sample. The sensitivity of PCR for detecting *C. albicans* organisms added to whole blood was 100 CFU/0.5 mL. In contrast, using the same spiked whole blood specimens, the lower limit of blood culture detection was approximately 10 CFU of *C. albicans* per 0.5 mL of blood.

Study Sample PCR and Blood Culture Results

Of the 70 samples from which DNA was extracted, 13 were associated with a positive blood culture for fungus. Nine of the thirteen positive cultures yielded *Candida* species, of which six were *C. albicans*, one *C. glabrata*, and two mixed *C. albicans* and *C. krusei*. All nine *Candida* culture-positive samples were positive by 18s rRNA PCR. The remaining four positive blood cultures yielded *Malassezia furfur*, and of these, only one was positive by fungal PCR. This PCR-positive patient was classified as high index of suspicion for septicemia. In contrast, the three patients whose blood cultures yielded *M. furfur* but whose fungal PCR was negative had a low index of suspicion for sepsis.

Of the 57 blood samples negative for fungal growth by culture, thirteen (23%) were PCR positive for 18s rRNA (positive predictive value 43%). Of the thirteen PCR positive/culture negative patients, seven had evidence of possible invasive fungal infection (Table 1). Four patients were being treated with amphotericin B for previous candidemia (3, 14, 24, and 28 days prior to study sample collection). Two neonates had *Candida albicans* isolated from urine obtained from a suprapubic bladder tap. Both of these patients were classified as high index of suspicion for sepsis and had no other positive cultures. One patient had necrotizing enterocolitis with intestinal perforation and *Candida* peritonitis at the time of study sample collection. In contrast, of the 44 samples that were both fungal PCR and culture negative, no patient had evidence of invasive fungal disease. Of the fifteen blood samples from healthy adults, two (13%) were positive for fungal DNA by 18s rRNA PCR.

Table 1. Characteristics of patients with positive PCR and negative blood culture for fungus

Unit	Index of Suspicion*	Clinical factors	Antifungal therapy	Relevant cultures
NICU	High	NEC	Completed amphotericin B course 14 days prior	Blood: C. albicans 28 days prior to sample collection.
NICU	High		On amphotericin	Blood: C albicans 3, 5 and 8 days prior to sample collection.
NICU	High	NEC, intestinal perforation	–	Blood: Enterococcus faecalis Peritoneal fluid: Klebsiella Blood: C glabrata 28 days prior to sample collection
NICU	High		On amphotericin	Blood: C. albicans 14 days prior to sample collection.
NICU	High		–	Urine: C albicans
NICU	High		–	Urine: C. albicans 4 days after study sample collection
NICU	High	NEC, intestinal perforation	–	Peritoneal fluid: Heavy C. albicans 4 days after study sample collection
NICU	High		–	Blood: Klebsiella pneumoniae
NICU	High	NEC	–	Blood : Enterobacter cloacae
PICU	High	ARDS, endocarditis	–	Blood: pseudomonas aeruginosa Sputum: heavy C.albicans, many PMNs
NICU	Moderate	Wrist abscess	–	Abscess fluid: pseudomonas aeruginosa.
NICU	Moderate		–	Blood: Staphylococcus epidermidis
NICU	Low		–	None.

* Index of suspicion for septicemia at the time of sample collection

In summary, compared with conventional blood culture, 18s rRNA PCR had 77% sensitivity, 77% specificity, 43% positive predictive value and 94% negative predictive value for detection of fungemia. Sensitivity and negative predictive value for detection of candidemia was 100%. If the seven cases of suspected disseminated *Candida* infection and the nine cases of blood culture proven infection are combined, the positive predictive value of this PCR for detection of disseminated *Candida* infection increases to 73% and its specificity to 88%.

Discussion

In hospitalized neonates and children, *Candida* is a leading cause of nosocomial sepsis, with significant mortality and morbidity (1,4,6). Early detection and aggressive treatment of disseminated *Candida* infection has been shown to decrease mortality, yet blood culture is suboptimal for rapid and sensitive detection of invasive fungal disease. In this study, we have shown that in NICU and PICU patients with suspected sepsis, 18s rRNA PCR can rapidly detect fungal DNA in all whole blood samples from which *Candida* was isolated by blood culture and may detect subclinical or low level candidemia.

This is the largest clinical study to date using PCR to detect fungemia in critically ill neonates and children. In blood volumes as small as 0.2 mL, 18s rRNA PCR was 100% sensitive for detection of blood culture-proven candidemia. Our findings are similar to those of the only other published neonatal/ pediatric study, in which Jordan et. al. performed PCR for the chitin synthase gene to detect *Candida* DNA in 26 of 27 paired blood samples from 16 patients with culture-proven candidemia (20). In contrast to the high sensitivity for detection of candidemia, sensitivity of our assay for detecting culture-proven *Malassezia furfur* was only 25%. Although *M. furfur* DNA can be amplified with the 18s rRNA primers used in this study (16,18), clinical studies have not demonstrated the ability of 18s rRNA PCR to detect septicemia with this relatively low-virulence yeast. In our study, the patient in whom PCR was positive and blood culture grew *M. furfur* was classified as high index of suspicion for septicemia, whereas the three patients in whom culture was positive and PCR negative had a low suspicion for sepsis. This suggests that our DNA extraction and PCR protocol may not be optimal for detection of low colony count *M. furfur* in the blood.

In vitro, the lower limits of sensitivity of our 18s rRNA PCR was 45 picograms of purified *C. albicans* DNA, which represents approximately 100 *Candida* organisms. The lower limit of detection of *C. albicans* organisms added to whole blood was also100 CFU per 0.5 ml. These results are comparable to other similar studies (20–23), although higher sensitivity has been reported using larger volumes of blood (18), nested PCR (19,24), and DNA hybridization of PCR products (16,18). In vivo studies in animal models have shown PCR to have equal or greater sensitivity than blood culture for *in vivo* detection of candidemia. In a neutropenic mouse model, Deventer et. al. demonstrated that whole blood 18s rRNA PCR followed by hybridization was more sensitive than blood culture for detection of experimental *C. albicans* bloodstream infection – 100% versus 67% sensitivity – (25). In the same study, PCR did not detect *Candida* DNA in the blood of colonized but noninfected animals. Similarly, nested PCR has been reported to be more sensitive than blood culture for detection of candidemia in an immunocompetent rabbit model (24,26). In humans, it has been estimated that a single blood culture, even by the lysis centrifugation method, fails to detect 25–50% of disseminated candidiasis (27). This leads us to speculate that some of the "false positive PCR" results in our study may actually represent false negative blood cultures in patients with disseminated fungal infection. PCR may be able to detect low colony count infection, intracellular or non-viable organisms, or free *Candida* DNA following clearance of the pathogen. The majority of patients (7 of 13) with positive PCR and negative culture had concurrent or prior evidence of possible invasive fungal disease, including two neonates with candiduria, strong clinical indicators of septicemia, and no other positive cultures, and one neonate with necrotizing enterocolitis, intestinal perforation and *C. albicans* peritonitis. Given that *Candida* colonization of the gastrointestinal tract and candiduria are strong predictors of systemic fungal infection (28–30), these three patients may have had disseminated *Candida* infection that was not detected by a single blood culture. Four PCR positive/culture negative patients had previous blood culture-proven candidemia from 3 to 28 days prior to sample collection and had received amphotericin treatment. Other investigators have also demonstrated persistence of positive fungal PCR for several weeks in a subgroup of patients on appropriate therapy for candidemia whose blood cultures had cleared (16,17).

Use of PCR for detection of disseminated fungal infection has a number of limitations. A positive PCR could indicate disseminated, life-threatening infection, transient fungemia which will clear without therapy, or contamination. In our healthy adult control group, the blood of two of fifteen individuals was positive for fungal DNA. While it is possible that immunocompetent individuals experience transient fungemia that is detectable by PCR, these results may also represent contamination during sample collection or processing. Even under stringent assay conditions, fungal PCR contamination rates of 18–35% have been reported in literature (17,18). This highlights the fact that fungal PCR will only be useful in combination with cultures and clinical acumen for determining which high-risk patients are likely to have disseminated fungal infection.

Prompt detection and treatment of disseminated fungal infection remains a challenge to clinicians caring for critically ill neonates and children. A rapid and reliable diagnostic test would not only improve outcome for patients with fungemia but also reduce the morbidity associated with empiric antifungal therapy for those who are not infected. Our data suggests that 18s rRNA PCR may be more sensitive than blood culture for detection of *Candida* sepsis. With further studies to determine the significance of positive PCR results when blood cultures are negative, PCR may ultimately prove to be a useful adjunct to blood culture for the rapid detection of life-threatening disseminated fungal infections.

References

1 Butler KM, Baker CJ. Candida: an increasingly important pathogen in the nursery. *Pediatr Clin North Am.* 1988;35:543–563

2. Stamos JK, Rowley AH. Candidemia in a pediatric population. *Clin Infect Dis.* 1995;20:571–575

3. Viscoli C, Girmenia C, Marinus A, et al. Candidemia in cancer patients: a prospective, multicenter surveillance study by the Invasive Fungal Infection Group (IFIG) of the European

Organization for Research and Treatment of Cancer (EORTC). *Clin Infect Dis.* 1999;28:1071–1079

4. Saiman L, Ludington E, Pfaller M, et al. Risk factors for candidemia in Neonatal Intensive Care Unit patients. The National Epidemiology of Mycosis Survey study group. *Pediatr Infect Dis J.* 2000;19:319–324
5. Stoll BJ, Gordon T, Korones SB, et al. Late-onset sepsis in very low birth weight neonates: a report from the National Institute of Child Health and Human Development Neonatal Research Network. *J Pediatr.* 1996;129:63–71
6. Kossoff EH, Buescher ES, Karlowicz MG. Candidemia in a neonatal intensive care unit: trends during fifteen years and clinical features of 111 cases. *Pediatr Infect Dis J.* 1998;17:504–508
7. Faix RG. Invasive neonatal candidiasis: comparison of albicans and parapsilosis infection. *Pediatr Infect Dis J.* 1992;11:88–93
8. Benjamin DK, Ross K, McKinney RE, Auten R, Fisher RG. When to suspect fungal infection in neonates: A clinical comparison of Candida albicans and Candida parapsilosis fungemia with coagulase-negative staphylococcal bacteremia. *Pediatrics.* 2000;106:712–718
9. Yamamura DL, Rotstein C, Nicolle LE, Ioannou S. Candidemia at selected Canadian sites: results from the Fungal Disease Registry, 1992–1994. Fungal Disease Registry of the Canadian Infectious Disease Society. *Cmaj.* 1999;160:493–499
10. Johnson DE, Thompson TR, Green TP, Ferrieri P. Systemic candidiasis in very low-birth-weight infants (less than 1,500 grams). *Pediatrics.* 1984;73:138–143
11. Pacheco-Rios A, Avila-Figueroa C, Nobigrot-Kleinman D, Santos JI. Mortality associated with systemic candidiasis in children. *Arch Med Res.* 1997;28:229–232
12. Fraser VJ, Jones M, Dunkel J, et al. Candidemia in a tertiary care hospital: epidemiology, risk factors, and predictors of mortality. *Clin Infect Dis.* 1992;15:414–421
13. Dato VM, Dajani AS. Candidemia in children with central venous catheters: role of catheter removal and amphotericin B therapy. *Pediatr Infect Dis J.* 1990;9:309–314
14. Eppes SC, Troutman JL, Gutman LT. Outcome of treatment of candidemia in children whose central catheters were removed or retained. *Pediatr Infect Dis J.* 1989;8:99–104
15. BaleyJE, Kliegman RM, Fanaroff AA. Disseminated fungal infections in very low birth weight infants: clinical manifestations and epidemiology. *Pediatrics.* 1984;73:144–152
16. Einsele H, Hebart H, Roller G, et al. Detection and identification of fungal pathogens in blood by using molecular probes. *J Clin Microbiol.* 1997;35:1353–1360
17. Hebart H, Loffler J, Reitze H, et al. Prospective screening by a panfungal polymerase chain reaction assay in patients at risk for fungal infections: implications for the management of febrile neutropenia. *Br J Haematol.* 2000;111:635–640
18. Van Burik JA, Myerson D, Schreckhise RW, Bowden RA. Panfungal PCR assay for detection of fungal infection in human blood specimens. *J Clin Microbiol.* 1998;36:1169–1175
19. Chryssanthou E, Andersson B, Petrini B, Lofdahl S, Tollemar J. Detection of Candida albicans DNA in serum by polymerase chain reaction. *Scand J Infect Dis.* 1994;26:479–485
20. Jordan JA. PCR identification of four medically important Candida species by using a single primer pair. *J Clin Microbiol.* 1994;32:2962–2967
21. Buchman TG, Rossier M, Merz WG, Charache P. Detection of surgical pathogens by in vitro DNA amplification. Part I. Rapid identification of Candida albicans by in vitro amplification of a fungus-specific gene. *Surgery.* 1990;108:338–46
22. Holmes AR, Cannon RD, Shepherd MG, Jenkinson HF. Detection of Candida albicans and other yeasts in blood by PCR. *J Clin Microbiol.* 1994;32:228–231
23. Miyakawa Y, Mabuchi T, Fukazawa Y. New method for detection of Candida albicans in human blood by polymerase chain reaction. *J Clin Microbiol.* 1993;31:3344–3347
24. Bougnoux M, Dupont C, Mateo J et al. Serum is more suitable than whole blood for diagnosis of systemic candidiasis by nested PCR. *J Clin Microbiol.* 1999;37:925–930
25. van Deventer AJM, Goessens WHF, van Belkum A, van Vliet HJA, van Etten EWM and Verbrugh HA. Improved detection of Candida albicans by PCR in blood of neutropenic mice with systemic candidiasis. *Journal of Clinical Microbiol.* 1995;33:625–628

26. Polanco A, Mellado E, Castilla C, Rodriguez-Tudela JL. Detection of Candida albicans in blood by PCR in a rabbit animal model of disseminated candidiasis. *Diagn Microbiol Infect Dis.* 1999;34:177–183
27. Berenguer J, Buck M, Witebsky F, Stock F, Pizzo PA, Walsh TJ. Lysis-centrifugation blood cultures in the detection of tissue-proven invasive candidiasis. Disseminated versus single-organ infection. *Diagn Microbiol Infect Dis.* 1993;17:103–109
28. Phillips JR, Karlowicz MG. Prevalence of Candida species in hospital-acquired urinary tract infections in a neonatal intensive care unit. *Pediatr Infect Dis J.* 1997;16:190–194
29. Calandra T, Bille J, Schneider R, Mosimann F, Francioli P. Clinical significance of Candida isolated from peritoneum in surgical patients. *Lancet.*1989;2:1437–1440
30. Solomkin JS, Flohr AB, Quie PG, Simmons RL. The role of Candida in intraperitoneal infections. *Surgery.* 1980;88:524–530

National Winner

A New Approach Of Endotoxin Testing By Using A Monoclonal Antibody Against Endotoxin (WN1-222/5) And Flow Cytometry

J. Nolde[1], F. E. Di Padova[2], H. Brade H.[3], K. H. Staubach[1]

[1] Dept. Surgery, Medical University of Luebeck, Luebeck, GERMANY
[2] Novartis, Basel, SWITZERLAND
[3] Forschungszentrum Borstel, Medical University of Luebeck, Luebeck, GERMANY

Abstract

Introduction

The limulus amoebocyte lysate (LAL) test has been used to indicate the presence of endotoxin in plasma for many years. Discordant results were explained by variations in preparation, lack of sensitivity but also specifity of the test assay.

In 1993 Di Padova and colleagues were able to generate a broadly cross-reactive monoclonal antibody (Mab) Wn1-222/5 recognizing the core region of E.coli, Shigella and salmonella R- and S-form LPS. Since Wn1-222/5 is capable of recognizing the immunogenic and antigenic epitope, it can be used in a therapeutical as well as in a diagnostic way.

Methods

Assay procedure

Heparinized blood samples were drawn into pyrogen-free vacutainer tubes from an peripherial arterial line. All following preparations were done at 4°C. Porcine mononuclear cells (MNC) were purified by dextran sedimentation and centrifugation at 1200 x g on 10 mL Ficoll-Paque (Pharmacia, Sweden). Erythrocytes were lysed with buffered ammonium chloride. The remaining MNCs were washed twice (10 and 5 minutes) and resuspended in PBS.

In order to measure endotoxin, 2×10^6 MNCs were fixed in 1 mL PFA 2%, washed and permeabilized by 1 mL sterile and pyrogen-free saponin solution 0.5% and incubated with 1 µl WN1-222-5 for 20 minutes. The samples were washed once again and then resuspended in 0.5 ml PBS. The samples were then incubated for 20 minutes in the dark with a fluorescent antibody Goat anti-mouse IgG 2a (M32204 Medac, Hamburg), washed again and fixed in 1mL PFA 2%.

As a negative control measurement all experiments were also performed with an iso-antibody IgG2a (Phar, Mingen).

Measurement was performed using a flow cytometer (FACScan, Becton Dickinson) by the red excitation-light (PE) of 585 nm with an argon-ion laser. During data acquisition (CellQuest-Software, Becton Dickinson) a "live" gate was set in the red fluorescence histogram. Mean fluorescence and the relation of positive cells compared to the iso-antibody were obtained as a correlation to the amount of endotoxin per defined amount of MNCs. Final mean fluorescence values (see Fig. 1 and 2) result from the diffrence of Wn1-fluorescence subtracted by the corresponding Iso-antibody values.

Porcine shock mode

Ten mechanically ventilated pigs received under analgosedation with fentanyl (0.01mg/kgBW/h), midazolam (0.1mg/kg BW/h) and pancuronium (0.1mg/kg BW/h) a continuous endotoxin infusion of salmonella fridenau (1µg/kg BW/h) until they succumed. Blood samples were drawn at baseline, after 1, 4 and 8 hours of the experiment. Assay preparation were done as mentioned under a).

In-vitro Measurement

To evaluate the diagnostic range of Wn1-222/5 blood samples were incubated 30min under 37°C with increasing amounts (see Fig. 1) of *Salmonella fridenau*, either with 10^6 MNCs and 5ml of porcine blood-serum from the same pig (Serum-incubation) or 5ml of heparinized whole-blood samples (Whole-blood incubation). Assay preparation were done as mentioned under a).

Wn1-222/5 Antibody

Wn1 binds to the five known E.coli core chemotypes, to Salmonella core, and to S-form LPS having these core structures. In immunoblots, it is shown to react with both the nonsubstituted core LPS and with LPS carrying O-side chains, indicating the exposure of the epitope in both S-form and R-form LPS. This Mab is not lipid A reactive but binds to E.coli J5, an RcP+ mutant which carries an inner core structure common to many members of the family *Enterobacteriaceae*. Phosphate groups present in the inner core contribute to the epitope but are not essential for the binding of WN1 to complete core LPS. WN1 222-5 binds to all E.coli clinical isolates tested so far and to some Citrobater, Enterobacter, and Klebsiella isolates.

Results

The in-vitro measurements were summarized in Figure 1a) and b).

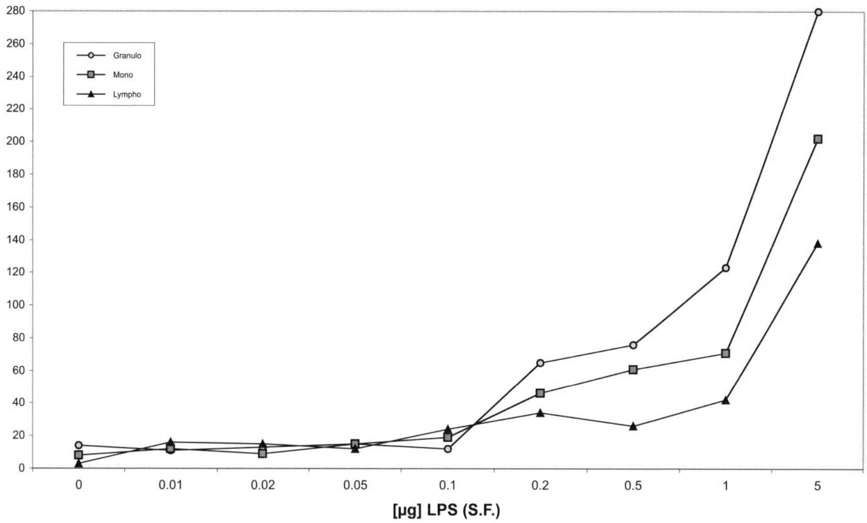

Figure 1a. whole-blood Incubation

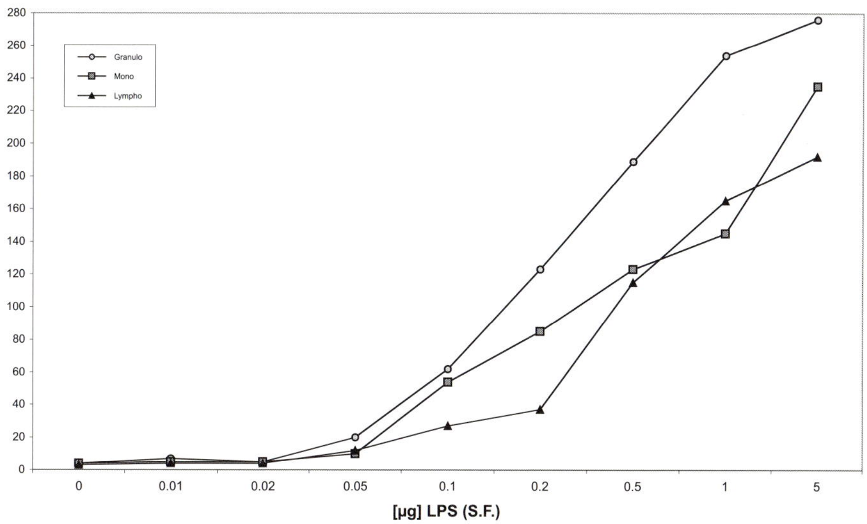

Figure 1b. blood-serum Incubation

The in-vivo results are shown in Table 1.

Table 1. Mean fluorescence as a function of hours of endo-toxin challenge

Hours of endo toxin challenge	Mean fluorescence		
	PNs	Mos	Lymph
0	22.3	14.3	8.43
1	82.4	24.5	17.7
4	76.6	193.0	81.3
8	72.4	175.0	76.1

Conclusions:

The OMNs reveal their highest activity to inernalize endotoxin initially in contrast to monocytes and lymphocytes which reached their summit at 4 hours. Thereafter all 3 cell lines keeep their internalzation rate high. At baseline endotoxin internalization of PMNs is already twice as high as in monocytes and lympohcytes. The in-vivo procedure in contrast to the in-vitro test data could not detect any endotoxin at the cell surface. In the proposed new blood endotoxin test assay with a cross-reactive endotoxin Mab a specific kinetic internalization of endotoxin in different cell lines could be found.

ORGANIZATIONAL ASPECTS

National Winner

Improvement Of Critical Care Management In A Healthcare Area By Implementing Point-Of-Care Testing In Primary Care. A Preliminary Approach

M. L. Hortas[1], I. Pérez-Montaut[2], M. Redondo[1], N. Montiel[1], R. Molina[3], C. González[1]

[1] Clinical Laboratories. Costa del Sol Hospital. Marbella. Málaga. SPAIN.
[2] Emergency Department. Las Lagunas Health Centre. Costa del Sol Primary Care. Mijas. SPAIN.
[3] Emergency Department. Costa del Sol Hospital. Marbella. SPAIN.

Abstract

Introduction

Because of computer-based data processing, a revolution in laboratories organisation has occurred. Consequently, diagnostic tools have been removed from Primary Care (PC) centres as laboratories were incorporated into hospitals. We are currently developing a project to promote the attendance of critically ill patients in primary care as first step in our healthcare system, in order to reduce derivation of patients to hospital emergency rooms. The aim of this study is to design and evaluate a model of analytical support to be provided to emergency departments in PC.

Methods

As a part of an overall project to ensure Point of Care Testing (POCT) quality in the Healthcare Area, this study will analyse the following steps: (1) implementation of new tests in PC; (2) devices criteria selection; (3) analytical quality control design; (4) elaboration of a guide to standard proceedings for performance of each test and quality control; (5) staff training to apply devices; and (6) organisational proposal for point of care service and its impact on central laboratory management and on hospital and PC emergency procedures.

Results

Preliminary results reveals that analytes suitable to be implemented in Costa del Sol PC emergency departments are blood gases, troponin T and β-Ketones. Operationally, POC devices must be in good agreement with that of the central laboratoryn and be easy to use. However, it is necessary to define goals for quality control programme and to establish indicators to evaluate the quality of the project. The central laboratory must train staff to carry out the full program, even on weekends. Flow information is an essential step in POCT organisation; as connectivity is a crucial aspect of the success of the programme.

Conclusions

We believe that implementation of POCT will lead to a review of clinical protocols and thus better management and care provision for critical health cases. This clinical outcome will be accompanied by the application of laboratory quality standards, the provision of reliable analytical data and an improvement in hospital emergency departments efficiency in dealing with critically ill patients. Further studies are being conducted to define cost analysis and performance of the tests under quality standards.

MISCELLANEOUS

National Winners

Studies On The Potential Effect Of Nitrite

Y. Tian, C. Wang, S. Song

Department of Clinical Chemistry, Chinese PLA General Hospital, Beijing, China

Abstract

Introduction

Extensive studies have been conformed that nitric oxide (NO) can elicit many of the various physiological regulatory functions including smooth muscle relaxation as endothelium-derived relaxing factor (EDRF) (1) and it is also well know that NO is very easy to be oxidized to nitrite/nitrate under physiological condition. Our previous studies indicated that nitrite could react with reduced thiols at low pH condition to form S-nitrosothiols which is responsible for vasodilation (2). The results conduct us to get a hypothesis that "nitrite is a modulator of vasodilation by forming S-nitrosothiols at low pH" and the propures of this studies is to conform that nitrite could initiate the depression of blood pressure.

Methods

Ten New Zealand white rabbits were used as animal model and their blood pressure continuously monitored by Helligeli electrophysiological monitor. The blood gas and methemoglobin(metHb) were also measured by an AVL analyzer. The blood nitrite were measured using Griess reagents.

Results

Animal experiment indicated that blood pressure was significantly depressed in concentration dependent manner after nitrite was infused intravenously to New Zealand white rabbits (Figure1). About 3 minutes, the blood drop to the lowest level and then gradually increased. At the mean time, the blood gas and metHb were no obvious changes after the nitrite was infused.

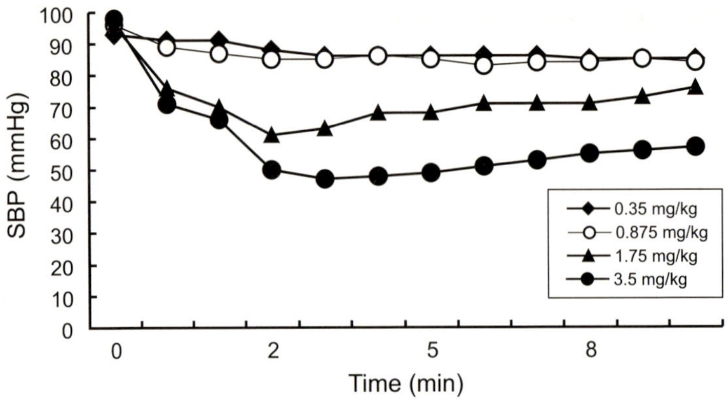

Figure 1. Nitrite depress SBP concentration dependently

Conclusions

The presence of nitrite in the human body has been well-documented (3), and it is believed to be either a product of normal metabolism or a direct result of food intake and bacterial product. Our previous studies had found that organic nitrate vasodilation drug was usually initiated the increasing of blood nitrite. These studies further confirm that nitrites themselves are vasodilator which may have the potential possibility as the bio-marker of vasodilation process. Further studies will be carrying out.

References

1 Murad-F. Discovery of some of the biological effects of nitric oxide and its role in cell signaling.Biosci Rep 1999; 19: 133–154

2. Tian YP, Rokicinski M and Betts WH, Nitrite may be an important EDRF modulator, Acta Biochimica et Biophysica Sinica 1999; 31:133–137

3. Eisenbrand, G, Spiegelhalder, B. and Preussmann, R., Nitrate and nitrite in saliva. Oncology 1980; 37: 227-231

Evaluation Of Some Laboratory Abnormalities In Acute Opiate Intoxication

H. T. Hung

Bach Mai Hospital, Hanoi, VIETNAM

Abstract

Introduction

Acute opiate intoxication is a common daily experience in the emergency departments and intensive care units and account for many overdose deaths. In Vietnam, narcotics are available in the black market. Most of them are heroin and opium. Overdose mortality is very high among opiate users. Besides, acute opiate poisoning causes not only severe and fatal complications during the time of hospitalization but also permanent sequelae.

Laboratory findings are very useful for diagnosis, early recognizing fatal complications and effective management. Of the laboratory investigations, the toxicological findings are the most credible evidences, and the arterial blood gases (ABGs) guide the decision of requiring mechanical ventilation in the cases of acute pulmonary edema and aspiration. In addition, many complications, which result in deaths or severe consequences if not early managed, are only recognized by the laboratory tests. Some of these complications are acute renal failure resulted from acute rhabdomyolysis, electrolyte disturbances, hypoglycemia, metabolic acidosis caused by hypoperfusion, hypoxemia or renal failure.

However, there have been few researches systematically evaluating laboratory abnormalities in acute opiate overdose, their important roles in diagnosis as well as their usefulness in management. Hence, our study was designed to evaluate laboratory abnormalities in acute opiate intoxication, and their important roles in the diagnosis and the treatment of acute opiate intoxication.

Methods

Patients

Subjects in this study were 32 adult patients with acute opiate overdose admitted to the emergency department, the poison control center, and the intensive care units in Bach Mai Hospital from 4-1999 to 4-2001.

Biochemical tests

- Blood specimens: glucose, electrolyte, BUN, creatinine, creatine kinase (CK), isoenzyme CK-MB, GOT, GPT, protein, albumin, A/G ratio, bilirubin, cholesterol, fibrinogen, prothrombin time, and HIV test.
- Urine specimens: protein, urea, and creatinine.

Hematological tests

Complete blood count (CBC)

Toxicological tests

- Urine specimens:
  The presence of opiates was determined by enzyme immunoassay (CIBA-CORNING Express Plus, CHIRON).
  Tests for 6-aminoacetyl morphine (6-MAM) in urine samples were done by thin-layer chromatography for patients suspected heroin overdose.
- Blood specimens:
  Morphine and 6-MAM were analyzed in blood samples by thin-layer chromatography.
- Gastric fluid specimens:
  Thin-layer chromatography was performed in cases of opiate ingestion.

Results

There were 4 patients with elevated uremia (> 7.5 mmoL/l) (12.5%). Their levels of serum creatinine were also high (> 120 mmol/L). All of them suffered from acute renal failure resulted from rhabdomyolysis. Hyperkalemia ($K^+ > 5$ mmol/l) were observed in 3 cases (9.4%). Particularly, one patient had very high level of serum potassium (7.3 mmol/L) at admission.

Fivecases (15.6%) with rhabdomyolysis (CK > 1000 UI/L) required forced diuretic and/or dialysis, and four of them developed acute renal failure.

Hypoglycemia was recognized in one case (1,9 mmol/L). On the other hand, there were 4 cases with hyperglycemia. These patients had no medical history of diabetes mellitus previously. It was regrettable that they themselves were discharge without any investigations.

In 7 cases (21.9%), the transaminase levels were elevated indicating hepatocellular damage. 2 of these patients developed hepatic insufficiency manifested by reducing albumin synthesis (hypoalbuminaemia, reverse A/G ratio), the failure of synthesis of clotting factors, and raising serum bilirubin levels.

One case had very low level of serum protein (38.1 g/l) and albumin (19 g/l). He had clinical manifestations of severe pulmonary edema at presentation.

Two patients were positive for 6-MAM in blood samples. In 2 other overdose patients resulted from ingestion of opiates, all gastric fluid samples were positive for morphine, one for heroin.

HIV tests were positive in 5 out of 26 patients (15.6%).

Conclusions

Laboratory findings, especially biochemical and arterial blood gas tests, have important roles in the diagnosis and the early recognition of fatal complications in acute opiate intoxication. In addition, laboratory data are valuable in treatment of acute opiate poisoning. They supply information for making decisions of treatment, especially in severe complications such as rhabdomyolysis and pulmonary edema.

Adhesion Molecules In An In Vitro Model Of Graft Rejection

S. Markovič[1,2], H. Daxecker[2], Ì. Raab[2], A. Griesmacher[2], M. M. Müller[2]

[1] Institute of Medical Biochemistry, Clinical Center of Serbia, Višegradska Belgrade, YUGOSLAVIA

[2] Institute of Laboratory Diagnostics and Ludwig Boltzmann Institute for Cardiothoracic Research, Kaiser Franz Josef Hospital, Vienna, AUSTRIA

Abstract

Introduction

Among the different factors playing crucial roles in endothelial cell activation, cytokines such as interleukin-1 (IL-1), interleukin-6 (IL-6), tumor necrosis factor-α (TNF-α) and interferon-γ (IFN-γ) have been reported to demonstrate profound effects on this cell type. In this study we stimulated endothelial cells with a mixture of those cytokines (IL-1β, IL-2, IL-4, IL-6, IL-10, TNF-α and IFN-γ), which were found at an elevated level in sera of patients with acute phase graft rejection. Furthermore, cytokine treated endothelial cells were co-incubated with CsA in a final concentration (5 μg/mL), that can be found at peak levels in serum of patients receiving immunosuppressive therapy after organ transplantations. The influence of this drug on the surface expression of a number of adhesion molecules (i.e. ICAM-1, VCAM-1, E-selectin, P-selectin, PECAM-1 and the L-selectin ligand CD 34) was determined by means of FACS.

Methods

Endothelial cells were stimulated with a mixture of different cytokines. In addition, endothelial cells were co-incubated with CsA (10 μl of a 0.5 mg/mL ethanolic stock solution per ml medium giving a final concentration of 5 μg/mL). Surface expression of adhesion molecules (ICAM-1, VCAM-1, E-selectin, P-selectin, PECAM-1 and the L-selectin ligand CD 34) were measured after an incubation period of 16 hours.

Adhesion molecule expression was investigated via flow-cytometric experiments. Cellular samples were incubated with an excess of the specific antibody for 30 minutes at 4°C. The following cell surface antigens were determined via FACS analysis: E-selectin (FITC), CD 34 (PE), P-selectin (FITC), ICAM-1 (PE), VCAM-1 (FITC) and PECAM-1 (PE). MFI obtained for stimulated cells were compared with the MFI of unstimulated cells serving as control values. All incubation experiments were performed five times.

Results

Of the adhesion molecules investigated, E-selectin expression was influenced most significantly. After stimulation with cytokine mixture E-selectin expression was up-regulated to 805 ± 112%. Under concomitant stimulation with CsA, the E-selectin level was significantly down-regulated resulting in 679 ± 145% compared to control values. VCAM-1 surface expression was also statistically significantly influenced by the cytokines mixture used. Incubation of cells with the mixture mentioned above led to an increase in MFI to 648 ± 57%. Concomitant incubation of endothelial cells with cytokine mixture plus CsA significantly reduced VCAM-1 expression (358 ± 106%). All other cell surface molecules tested were not influenced to a comparable extent.

Conclusions

Our data showed that immunosuppression by CsA is also achieved by decreasing the expression of adhesion molecules on endothelial cells, which are the first target of the cellular rejection process. Our results clearly demonstrate that incubating cytokine stimulated endothelial cells with a final CsA concentration of 5 µg/mL had a significant down-regulating influence on the surface expression of E-selectin and VCAM-1.

Index

Symbols

18s ribosomal DNA 164
18s ribosomal RNA PCR 165
18s rRNA PCR 170
4G/5G polymorphism 66

A

Abciximab 122
ACR 52, 55, 58
ACTH 32, 37, 42
  in sepsis and multiple trauma 37
Acute ischemic stroke 111
Acute lung injury (ALI) 144
Acute respiratory distress syndrome (ARDS) 143
Acute stroke 111
Adhesion molecules 111, 192
  in acute stroke 111
  in endothelial cells 192
Adrenocortical axis 43
Adult respiratory distress syndrome 36, 58, 77, 143
  bronchoalveolar lavage 80
Adult respiratory distress syndrome (ARDS) 34
Albumin creatinine ratio, urine 52
ANP 115
APACHE II 55
Apoptosis 3, 4
  in sepsis and multiple organ dysfunction syndrome 3
ARDS 40, 43, 58, 77, 86
Arterial blood gases 189
Artificial heart valves 120
Assay 177

B

β-globin gene 146
  real time PCR 146
BAL 80
BAL subfractions 84
Blood culture 166
Blood pressure 187
BNP 116
Brain trauma 127
Bronchoalveolar lavage 80, 84
  subfractions 84
Bronchoalveolar lavage fluid 80
Burns 51

C

C-reactive protein in IBD 158
Candida albicans 164
  culture, blood culture sensitivity, PCR 166
Candida DNA by polymerase chain reaction (PCR) 165
Candida DNA extraction 167
Candida infection 164
Capillary permeability 49
Cardiac troponin T (cTnT) 97, 102
CART analysis 149
Cell adhesion molecules (CAM) 111
Chron's disease 159
CK 160
CK-MB 99

CK-MB mass 99
CMV 69
  hybrid capture DNA assay 69
CMV-DNA 69
Concentration in serum 132
Cortisol 32, 37
  in sepsis and multiple trauma 37
Creatine kinase (CK)
  in duchenne muscular dystrophy 160
Creatine kinase MB 99
  mass, peak concentration in myocardial infarction 99
CRP 17, 23, 25, 37, 137, 159
  in inflammatory bowel disease 159
  in sepsis and multiple trauma 37
  in sepsis and septic shock 37
Cystatin C 115
  in hemodialysis 115
Cytokines 10, 33, 42, 192
  in sepsis and mutiple organ dysfunction syndrome 10

D

DHEAS 32
Dialysis 115
Disseminated intravascular coagulation 65, 121, 159
Diuresis 116
DMD 159
DNA extraction 166
Duchenne muscular dystrophy 159

E

Endothelial cells 192
Endothelium-derived relaxing factor (EDRF) (1) 187
Endotoxin 177
  assay 177
Estimate the infarct size 97

F

Fas-ligand 11
Flow cytometer 178
Flow-cytometric 192
Flowcytometry 177, 192
  adhesion molecules 192
  limulus amoebocyte lysate test 177
Functional polymorphism 66
Fungal infections 163
Fungal species 163

G

Gated SPECT 105
GC 43
Glucocorticoids 33

H

Haptoglobin 72
  polymorphism in tuberculosis 72
Haptoglobin polymorphism 72
Healthy 157
Hemodiafiltration 116
HIV 70
HIV-1 RNA 71
HIV-RNA 70
HPA 41
Hypocalcemia 29
  in septic shock 29
Hypothalamo-pituitary-adrenal function 32
Hypothalamus-pituitary-adrenal (HPA) axis 34

I

IBD 157
IL-6 37, 42
IL-6, IL-8, and IL-10 7
Illness severity scores 57
Immuno-Polymerase Chain Reaction (Immuno-PCR) 156
Immunoassay procedures S100BB 130
Immunocompromised patients 69
Immunosuppressive therapy 192
Infarct size 102
Inflammatory bowel diseases (IBD) and Duchennne mu 154, 157

Interleukin-6 37
 in sepsis and multiple trauma 37
Ionized calcium (Ca2+) 17, 21
 in sepsis 21
 Mc Lean-Hastings equation 20

L

LBP 37, 42
Left ventricular ejection fraction (LVEF) 103
Leucocyte count 17
Limulus amoebocyte lysate (LAL) test 177
Lipoprotein-binding-protein 32, 37
 in sepsis and multiple trauma 37
LOD score 5
Lung surfactant 77
LV ejection fractions (LVEF) 97, 105

M

Macrophage migration inhibitory factor (MIF) 32, 37, 42
 in sepsis and multiple trauma 37
Magnesium 93
 therapy in ICU-patients 93
Malignant lymphomas 119
Malignant melanoma 127
Mb 160
Mc Lean-Hastings equation 20
Mechanical heart valves 120
Meningococcaemia 65
Microalbuminuria 47, 48, 49, 58
MIF 37, 42
Mononuclear cells 177
Mortality probabilities 55
Multiple organ dysfunction syndrome (MODS) 3, 4
Multiple organ failure (MOF) 47
Multiple trauma 37
Multitrauma 32
Myocardial infarction 97, 101
 CK-MB mass 100
 SPECT imaging 101
 troponin T 101
Myocardial reperfusion 122
Myoglobin 160
 in Duchenne muscular dystrophy 160
Myoglobin (Mb) 160

N

Natriuretic peptides 115
Neurohumoral cytokine response 43
Nitric oxide (NO) 187
Nucleosome ELISA 6
Nucleosome plasma levels 8
Nucleosomes 3, 5, 6, 8, 11
 in plasma 8
 in sepsis 8

O

Opiate intoxication 189

P

PAF-acetylhydrolase (PAF-AcH) 77
PAI 1 65
 gene 66
PCR 146, 163
PCT 37
Peak concentrations 99
Perfusion defect 101
Phospholipase A2 79, 81, 83
 assay 81
Phospholipase A2 / PAF-AcH fluorimetric assay 81
Phospholipase A2 and PAF-acetylhydrolase levels in BAL 83
Phospholipases (PLases) A2 77
Phospholipases A2 and PAF-acetylhydrolase 86
Plasma β-globin DNA 147
Plasma DNA 142, 147
 β-globin 147
 in trauma, acute respiratory distress syndrome 143
Plasma PCT 25
 prognostic value 28
Plasminogen activator 122

Plasminogen activator inhibitor 1 65
  4G/5G polymorphism in meningococcaemia 65
Platelet glycoprotein IIb/IIIa inhibitor 122
Platelet-activating factor acetylhydrolase (PAF-AcH) 77, 79, 83
Point-of-care testing 183
Polymerase chain reaction 146, 163
  fungal species 163
  real time PCR, β globin gene 146
Predict infarct size and LV function in patients with AMI 105
Procalcitonin (PCT) 17, 18, 25, 26, 28, 37, 42
  in sepsis 17, 26
  in sepsis and multiple trauma 37
  prognostic value 28
Proteins 127
Purpura fulminans 65

R

Real time 146
Recombinant t-PA 122

S

S-100 family 127
S-100 protein 127, 129, 137
  assay 129
  in malignant melanoma and brain trauma 127
S-100A1B 127
S-100BB 127
S100B 128
  assay 137
S100BB 129
SAP II 55
Sepsis 4, 17
Septic shock 3, 5, 17, 22, 25, 32, 37, 43, 65
Serum lipid peroxides (PD) 122
Serum sTfR 119
Serum TNFα concentrations 157
sFas 11
SIRS 5
SOFA score 6
Soluble transferrin receptor 119
  in malignant lymphoma 119
SPECT imaging 99
Streptokinase 122
Systemic inflammatory response syndrome (SIRS) 47, 57

T

Thiobarbituric acid reactive substances (TBARS) 122
Thrombocytic hemostasis 120
TNF-α 11, 32, 37, 154, 156, 157, 159
  assay 156, 159
  in duchenne muscular dystrophy 159
  in inflammatory bowel disease 157
  in sepsis and multiple trauma 37
Trauma 32, 37, 43, 51, 142
Trauma patients 142
Troponin T 97
  estimation of myocardial infarct size 97
Tuberculosis 72
Tumor necrosis factor a (TNF-α) 154, 155

U

Ulcerative colitis 159
Urine albumin creatinine ratio (ACR) 49

V

Vascular-thrombocytic hemostasis 120
Viral genomes 69
Viral load 71

About Roche and the Roche Diagnostics Division

Headquartered in Basel, Switzerland, Roche is one of the world's leading innovation-driven healthcare groups. Its core businesses are pharmaceuticals and diagnostics. Roche is number one in the global diagnostics market, the leading supplier of pharmaceuticals for cancer and a leader in virology and transplantation. As a supplier of products and services for the prevention, diagnosis and treatment of disease, the Group contributes on a broad range of fronts to improving people's health and quality of life. Roche employs roughly 65,000 people in 150 countries. The Group has alliances and research and development agreements with numerous partners, including majority ownership interests in Genentech and Chugai. Roche's Diagnostics Division, the world leader in in-vitro diagnostics with a uniquely broad product portfolio, supplies a wide array of innovative testing products and services to researchers, physicians, patients, hospitals and laboratories world-wide.

For further information, please visit our websites www.roche.com and www.roche-diagnostics.com.

Printing: Mercedes-Druck, Berlin
Binding: Stein+Lehmann, Berlin